DATES IN INFECTIOUS DISEASES

DATES IN

INFECTIOUS DISEASES

EDITED BY H.S.J. LEE

The Parthenon Publishing Group
International Publishers in Medicine, Science & Technology

A CRC PRESS COMPANY
BOCA RATON   LONDON   NEW YORK   WASHINGTON, D.C.

Published in the USA by
The Parthenon Publishing Group
345 Park Avenue South, 10th Floor
New York, NY 10010, USA

Published in the UK and Europe by
The Parthenon Publishing Group
23–25 Blades Court
Deodar Road, London SW15 2NU, UK

**Library of Congress Cataloging-in-Publication Data
available on request**

British Library Cataloguing in Publication Data

Dates in infectious diseases. - (Landmarks in medicine series)
    1. Communicable diseases - History - Chronology 2. Infection
I. Lee, H. S. J.
616.9'09

ISBN 1-84214-1503

No part of this book may be reproduced in any form without permission from the publishers, except for the quotation of brief passages for the purposes of review.

Copyright © 2002 Parthenon Publishing Group
A CRC Press Company

Printed and bound by
Butler & Tanner Ltd, Frome and London, UK

Acknowledgement

The editor would like to acknowledge
The National Library of Medicine,
The World Health Organization
and The Nobel Foundation.

DATES IN INFECTIOUS DISEASES

Introduction

Modern understanding of infectious disease is based on the achievements and contributions of many doctors and scientists over many years. To appreciate the state-of-the-art as it exists today, it is helpful to know something of the background and history of the subject as it has developed over the last few centuries – and as the underlying scientific principles have become more fully understood and elucidated.

This volume records some of the key milestones in the development of understanding of infectious diseases that have taken place over the last millennium. Of course, although some notable contributions were made in earlier centuries, it is really only in the later years of the present millennium that advances in knowledge and practice become numerous and significant. Naturally, too, these advances are closely related to progress in other fields of medicine – and this fact is also reflected in the pages of the book.

The milestones listed here are indeed important ones but are by no means comprehensive. Readers will all have their own individual views of additional important events that should be recorded, and I would certainly welcome their suggestions for the next edition.

It is hoped that the milestones described will provide an interesting reference and aide-memoire to all those with an interest in infectious disease who would like to know more about its background and development.

Dates in Infectious Diseases — Dates in Antiquity

1500 BC — First known mention of dracunculiasis found in the Turin Papyrus. An Egyptian mummy from that time was shown to be infected with *Dracunculus medinensis*.

1157 BC — RAMSES V, ruler of Egypt, was disfigured and died from smallpox.

600 BC — First reference to leprosy in India.

430 BC — The plague of Athens. War with Sparta causes 200,000 people to flood into Athens, bringing plague with them, and led to the decline of the State. It has been suggested that the plague was a form of typhus.

400 BC — HIPPOCRATES thought that infection came from exposure to poisonous vapors from decaying living material. He provided the first record of an influenza pandemic in the year 412 BC. He identified phthisis (tuberculosis) and noted that it was almost always fatal.

212 BC — The Roman historian LIVY described an infectious disease resembling influenza, which affected the Roman army.

81 AD — ARETAEUS THE CAPPADOCIAN born. He described pulmonary tuberculosis, noted that the pulmonary tissue became insensitive to pain, and that chronic cough and hemoptysis were present, the nails became curved, the chest narrowed, there was weight loss, night sweats and pallor. He also gave an account of elephantiasis.

98 — RUFUS OF EPHESUS born. A Greek physician and surgeon who lived during the reign of the Emperor

Dates in Infectious Diseases

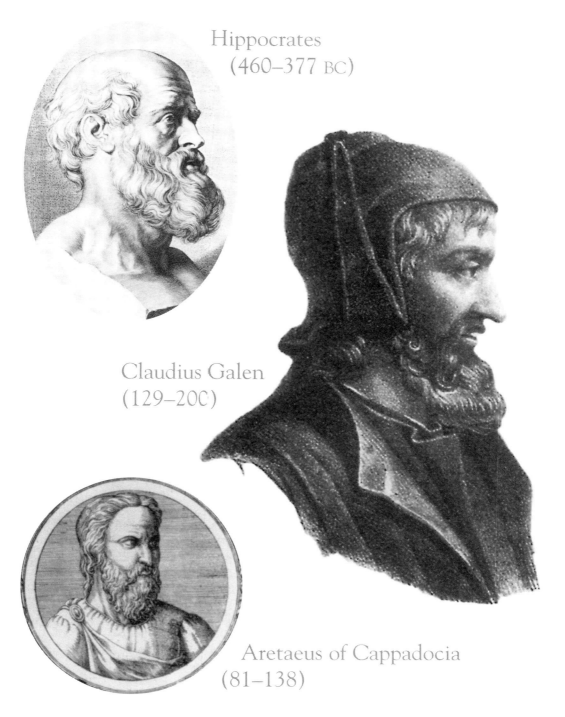

Hippocrates
(460–377 BC)

Claudius Galen
(129–200)

Aretaeus of Cappadocia
(81–138)

	Trajan, and gave a description of plague in his work *On Naming the Parts of the Body*.
125	Rome affected by anthrax that killed tens of thousands.
129	CLAUDIUS GALEN born in Pergamon in Asia Minor. He described the influence of the four humors and the three spirits on sickness and health, and introduced many drugs derived from plants. He was the first to describe smallpox.
160	Bubonic plague (Barbarian boils) caused the collapse of the Han Empire in China.
166	The Antonine plague (smallpox, measles and bubonic plague) reached Rome, killed Emperor MARCUS AURELIUS, and spread through the Empire, killing 4–7 million people in Europe and resulting in the fall of the Roman Empire.
314	The Church ordered regulations against lepers at the Council of Ancyra, defining lepers as bodily and morally unclean.
500	The Brahmin physician SUSRUTA is credited with first associating malaria with the mosquito.
540	A major plague epidemic occurred at Pelusium, Egypt, reached Constantinople in 542 and spread into Europe and Asia (the Plague of Justinian) in the following decade.
570	Bishop MARIUS OF AVENCHES was the first to use the term 'variola' (from 'varus', a pimple or tubercule) for smallpox.

777 — MESUE SENIOR born. An Arab physician, known to Latin Europe as JANUS DAMESCENUS, whose works included the *Mesue Opera*, illustrated with pictures of medicinal herbs, and *Book of Fevers*.

850 — RHAZES born. Great Arab physician who wrote *Al-Hawi*, which incorporated all medical, surgical, pharmacological and anatomical knowledge from Greece, Syria, India, Persia and the Roman Empire. His distinction between smallpox and measles led him to advocate the following treatment: 'All those pustules that are very large should be pricked; and the fluid that drops from them be soaked up with a soft clean rag in which there is nothing that may hurt or excoriate the patient'.

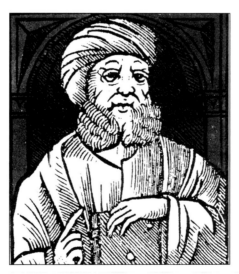

Rhazes (850–932)

980 — AVICENNA born in Chorassan, Persia. His *Al-Qanun Fil Tibba* consisting of five books, mentions dracunculiasis and gives detailed descriptions of the disease, treatment, and complications caused by the worm being ruptured during extraction.

Dates in Infectious Diseases

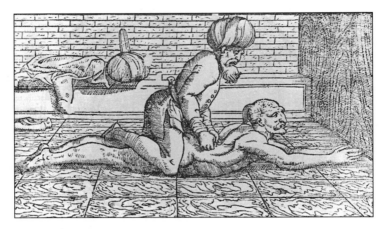

Avicenna administering massage (980–1037)

1104–10 Plague killed more than 90% of Europeans and, coincidentally, all those northern Europeans who were genetically predisposed to leprosy.

1179 The Third Lateran Council decreed that lepers should be identified and separated.

1180 GILBERTUS ANGLICUS born. An English medical writer who wrote *Compendium Medicinae*, mentioned sublimation and distillation and the use of red light in treatment of smallpox.

1329 ROBERT THE BRUCE of Scotland died of a mysterious ailment called the 'great malady', possibly leprosy. His skull was pitted and the upper jaw and nose eroded.

1345 A major plague epidemic started in the lower Volga River basin, reaching the Caucasus and Crimea in 1346, Constantinople in 1347, Alexandria, Cyprus and Sicily in 1347, Italy by winter 1347, Marseilles by January of 1348, Paris in spring 1348, followed by Germany, the Low Countries and England later that year, Norway in May 1349, eastern Europe by 1350, and finally Russia in 1351. Once it ebbed, it was estimated that one in three people were lost – a total of 40 million worldwide.

1347 Northern Italy introduced a temporary 40-day ban on travel and trade to control bubonic plague. This quarantine (from the Italian *quarentina*, meaning 40 days) was based on the number of days the Bible said Christ spent in the wilderness.

1348 The pope set up a commission of the medical faculty at Paris to investigate the cause of the Great Plague. They concluded that the disaster was a result of a conjunction of Saturn, Jupiter, and Mars in the 40th degree of Aquarius at 1:00 p.m. on March 20, 1345. This 'caused hot, moist conditions, which forced the earth to exhale a virulent sulfurous miasma'.

1478 GIROLAMO FRACASTORO born. An Italian physician from Verona who proposed a cause for infectious diseases in *De contagionibus*.

1489 Typhus was first identified at the siege of Granada.

1492 Introduction of influenza, smallpox, tuberculosis and gonorrhea to the Americas. Columbus' arrival in Hispaniola was followed by the death of eight million inhabitants. Slaves from Africa brought malaria and yellow fever which affected European settlers.

1493 PARACELSUS born. A physician, alchemist, philosopher and astrologer from Switzerland who was the founder of chemical therapeutics and introduced mercurials as treatment for syphilis. He coined the term 'French gonorrhea' in 1553 to denote syphilis, a terminology that created confusion between syphilis and gonorrhea for the next three centuries.

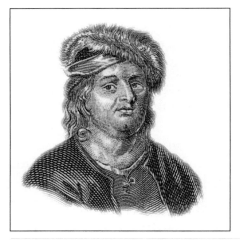

Paracelsus
(1494–1541)

1495 Syphilis reached Germany and Switzerland, then England and Holland in 1496. VASCO DA GAMA'S crew carried it around the Cape in 1497 causing an outbreak in India in 1498, which in turn spread eastward. China and Japan were affected in 1505.

1496 GIORGIO SOMMARIVA of Verona was the first person to use mercury to treat syphilis during the syphilis epidemic in Europe.

1498 The first Spanish treatise on syphilis was written by FRANCISCO LOPEZ DE VILLALOBOS, physician to King Charles I.

1500 THIERRY DE HERY born. A French physician who wrote a treatise on syphilis in which he recommended guaiacum resin to be taken internally, or mercury for injection or fumigation.

1506	JEAN FRANÇOIS FERNEL born. A French physician who published *Universa Medica* (a standard textbook for over a century), and was one of the first to treat gonorrhea and syphilis as two distinct diseases.
1510	First record of an epidemic of influenza in Europe.
1520	Smallpox was introduced to America by HERNANDO CORTEZ. 3,500,000 Aztecs died in the next two years.
1527	French physician JACQUES DE BETHENCOURT described syphilis as 'Morbus venereus'.
1530	Italian physician GIROLAMO FRACASTORO published *Syphilis, sive morbus Gallicus* (Syphilis, or the French disease). He suggested that this sexually transmitted disease was spread by 'seeds' distributed by intimate contact; he also said that the disease could be spread by something in the air. In the same year, he described rabies.
1539	An early account of neurosyphilis was given by Italian professor, NICCOLO MASSA.
1542	Bubonic plague from Egypt reached Constantinople and spread through Europe, killing 40% of the population.
c 1550	Measles and smallpox wiped out 95% of native South Americans. When CORTEZ took over Mexico City 1,000 Aztecs per day were dying.
1578	Whooping cough was described as 'tussis quintana' by Paris physician, GUILLAUME DE BAILLOU.

1589 Thomas Moffet gave the first description of living organisms causing disease when he identified lice, fleas and scabies mites.

1593 Fabricius Hildanus wrote a monograph on gangrene.

1607 Claude Tardi born. A French physician who proposed the theoretical basis for blood transfusion from man to man.

1609 Sanctorius invented the clinical thermometer.

1622 Richard Wiseman born. An orthopedic surgeon from Britain who described skeletal tuberculosis, wrote an important text entitled *Tumours* and made one of the first distinctions between tubercular and gonococcal arthritis.

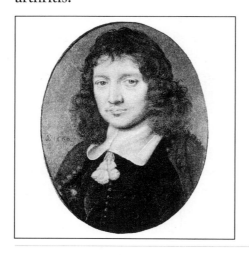

Richard Wiseman
(1622–1676)

1623 Trichuriasis, caused by an intestinal nematode parasite (*Trichura*), was described by Spanish physician, Alexo de Abreu.

1624	THOMAS SYDENHAM born. Sydenham has been described as the designer of modern clinical medicine and the 'English Hippocrates'. He treated rheumatic fever with 'moderate' bleeding, purgatives, bed rest and diet.
1626	FRANCESCO REDI born. An Italian physician from Arezzo credited with being the first parasitologist, who demonstrated that maggots developed from eggs laid by flies, and first described the reproductive process of the roundworm.
1627	An early monograph on fever was published by DANIEL SENNERT, professor of medicine at Wittenberg, Germany.
1630	In his posthumously published *Opera Medica*, FRANCISCUS SYLVIUS identified tubercles as a characteristic change in the lungs and other areas of consumptive patients. He also described their progression to abscesses and cavities.
1635	Yellow fever was reported in the Antilles by FATHER J.B. DUTERTRE.
1639	A landmark in therapeutics was the introduction of Cinchona bark as treatment for malaria by a Spanish physician, JUAN DEL VEGO.
1642	SIR ROBERT TABOR born. An apothecary from Cambridge who became famous through his secret remedy for malaria whose active ingredient was later found to be Cinchona bark, already in wide use as a cure for malaria.

1646	A treatise on plague was written by Dutch physician, ISBRAND VAN DIEMERBROCK.
1648	The first report of tropical dysentery in the East Indies was given by Leiden physician, JACOB DE BONTIUS. He wrote a book on tropical medicine, *Medicina Indorum*.
1658	ATHANASIUS KIRCHNER, a Jesuit priest from Germany, was the earliest to attempt to view microscopic organisms using a primitive microscope, and examined pus and red cells in plague victims. He suggested that micro-organisms cause infectious disease.
1659	THOMAS WILLIS, an English physician described epidemic typhoid fever, symptoms in achalasia cardia, headache, whooping cough and asthma in *De febribus*.

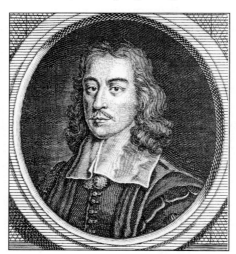

Thomas Willis
(1621–1675)

1661	THOMAS WILLIS wrote a report of cerebrospinal fever (meningitis) followed by a description six years later on the late-stage effects of syphilis on the brain in *Pathologiae cerebri*.

1665   NATHANIEL HODGES, a London physician who remained in the city during the plague epidemic, wrote an account, *Loimologia, or an Historical Account of the Plague in London*, giving symptoms, means of prevention and treatment.

1667   DANIEL TURNER born. A British physician regarded as the founder of dermatology who wrote an important treatise on syphilis.

1671   GEORGE CHEYNE born. A Scottish physician who wrote *A New Theory of Fevers* and *The English Malady or Treatise on Nervous Diseases*.

1672   FRANCIS CHICOYNEAU born. A French physician who advocated the theory that plague was not contagious, in a treatise he wrote after studies carried out during a plague epidemic in Marseilles.

1677   THOMAS THACHER wrote the first American pamphlet on smallpox, *A Brief Rule to Guide the Common People of New England how to order themselves and theirs in the Small Pocks, or Measles*.

1679   First mention of Yaws, a disease caused by *Treponema pallidum* ssp *pertenue* that occurs in warm, humid tropics.

1683   ANTON VAN LEEUWENHOEK used his microscope to observe and describe what he termed 'animacules', i.e. bacteria and protozoa from pond water and human saliva, and described the shapes of bacilli, cocci and spirilla bacteria.

Dates in Infectious Diseases

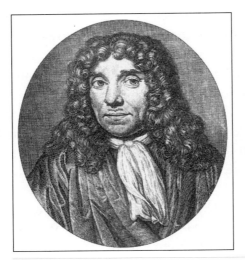

Anton van Leeuwenhoek (1632–1723)

1684 JEAN ASTRUC born. French physician in Paris, wrote a systematic treatise on syphilis, *De Morbis Veneris libri sex*. He considered that it originated in America and spread to Europe in 1493. His other works include *On the Inoculation of Small Pox*, *Origine de la Peste*, *De Mortu musculare*, and *The Diseases of Women*.

1684 London physician DAVID ABERCROMBY first suggested a parasitic cause for syphilis.

1686 A chronic tropical skin disease found in the Malay Archipelago and Southeast Asia (*Tinea imbricata*) was described in the Philippines by English navigator, SIR WILLIAM DAMPIER.

1687 GIOVANNI BONOMO and GIACENTO CESTONI of Italy established the mite *Acarus scabei* as the cause of scabies, the first time a microscopic organism had been established as the cause of a specific disease.

1701	Infection by germs as a cause of disease was proposed by French surgeon, NICHOLAS ANDRY.
1703	RICHARD MEAD reported to the Royal Society on 'the Worms of Humane Bodies'. 'Having frequently observed that the Poor Women when their Children are troubled with the Itch, do with the point of a Pin pull out of the Scabby Skin little Bladders of Water, and crack them like Fleas with their Nails ... it came to Mind to examine these Bladders ... I examined whether or no these Animalcules laid Eggs, and after many enquiries, at last good Fortune while I was drawing the Figure of one of 'em by a microscope, from the hinder part I saw drop a very small and scarcely visible white Egg.'
1706	BENJAMIN FRANKLIN born. An American scientist and statesman who invented the bifocal lens, pioneered the treatment of nervous diseases using electricity, and introduced inoculation for smallpox to America.
1707	CARL LINNAEUS, Swedish naturalist and physician, born. He was the first to suggest that dracunculiasis was caused by worms.
1710	WILLIAM HEBERDEN THE ELDER born. A London physician who described acute rheumatic fever, summer catarrh and asthma.
1711	A plague epidemic occurred in Austria.
1712	Italian physician, FRANCESCO TORTI introduced cinchona into Italy and coined the term 'mal aria' (bad air) for malaria in his *Therapeutica Specialis ad febres quasdam perniciosae*.

1717   GIOVANNI LANCISI of Rome wrote on influenza, cattle plague (rinderpest), and malaria. In his *De noxiis paludum effluvis* he made the connection between the prevalence of malaria in swampy districts to the presence of mosquitoes and recommended drainage of the swamps to prevent the disease.

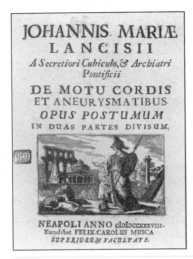

Frontispiece from one of Giovanni Maria Lancisi's books

1720   The last major outbreak of plague occurred in Marseilles.

1720   English physician BENJAMIN MARTEN, wrote *A New Theory of Consumption*, stating that tuberculosis could be caused by 'wonderfully minute living creatures' which generated the lesions.

1721   Variolation was introduced in England by LADY MARY MONTAGU for smallpox prevention. The technique was later refined by the Suttons. The method was first tried in England on seven condemned criminals. Later two members of the royal family were inoculated.

William Heberden the Elder
(1710–1801)

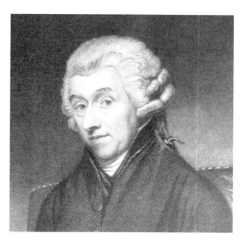

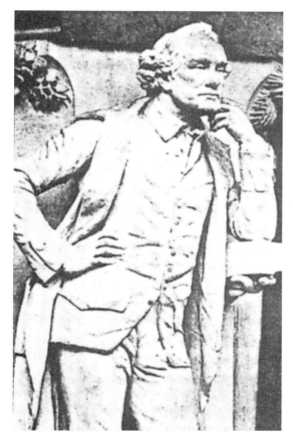

John Hunter
(1728–1793)

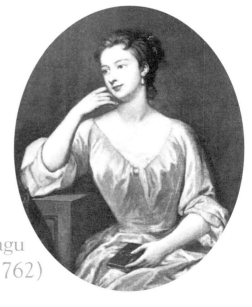

Lady Mary Wortley Montagu
(1689–1762)

1721	Outbreak of smallpox in Boston, and ZABDIEL BOYLSTON was the first to use inoculation in North America, where his son and two slaves were inoculated.
1724	Thirty per cent of the population of Williamsburg USA died of typhoid fever. Malaria had caused a move from Jamestown to Williamsburg.
1729	WILLIAM BUCHAN born. A Scottish physician who wrote *Domestic Medicine*, *Advice to Mothers* and *Treatise on Venereal Disease*.
1735	The first outbreak of 'throat distemper' (diphtheria) in America, in New Hampshire; it killed most of its child victims.
1736	JEAN ASTRUC of France published a paper on the contagious pathogenesis and infectious etiology of venereal diseases. He considered that venereal disease had come to Europe from America: 'In the Neapolitan, or rather in the Spanish, army there were not a few of the soldiers, who returning from the Indies, either in the first voyage of Christopher Columbus ... or in the second with Antonio de Torrez ... were as yet infected with the Venereal Disease, or at least had contracted it in Spain, after it had been brought by others into Europe'.
1739	FRANÇOIS QUESNAY, a surgeon in Paris, suggested an arterial cause for gangrene in his *Traite de la Gangrene*.
1747	GIOVANNI BATTISTA MORGAGNI, the founder of pathological anatomy from Forli in Italy, noted syphilitic tumors of the brain, tuberculosis of the kidney, and described the pathological changes in dysentery.

1756	A clinical description of leishmaniasis was provided by ALEXANDER RUSSELL, in a Turkish patient. The disease was commonly known as Aleppo boil.
1759	FRANCIS HOME, an Edinburgh physician, pioneered experimental inoculation against measles and published much of his work and research on measles, croup, diabetes and many other areas in *Medical Facts and Experiments*.
1760	PETER RUBINI born. An Italian physician from Parma who wrote several treatises on fever.
1761	GIOVANNI BATTISTA MORGAGNI published his three-volume *On the Sites and Causes of Disease*. He described syphilis, and refused to dissect any bodies with smallpox or tuberculosis. A tubercle is named after him.

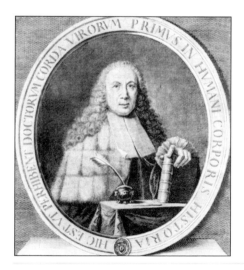

Giovanni Battista Morgagni (1682–1771)

1762	EUSEBIUS VALLI born. An Italian physician who tried the efficacy of plague vaccine on himself and survived, but succumbed to yellow fever in Cuba.

1767	Scottish surgeon, JOHN HUNTER inoculated himself with pus from a patient with gonorrhea to determine if the same cause existed for syphilis and gonorrhea. Unfortunately the patient had both diseases so Hunter maintained that they had the same infectious agent. In 1786, he described elevated papule in the penis or vulva seen in primary syphilis (Hunter chancre) and published *On Venereal Diseases*.
1768	ROBERT WHYTT, a Scottish professor, wrote on tuberculous meningitis in children in *Observations on Dropsy of the Brain*, and described hydrocephalus due to tuberculous meningitis (Whytt disease).
1770	A plague epidemic, lasting two years, occurred in the Balkans.
1771	JOHANN GEORG ZIMMERMANN from Switzerland, published a monograph on bacillary dysentery.
1776	THOMAS DIMSDALE, an English physician, wrote a treatise on smallpox inoculation, *Thought on General and Partial Inoculation*.
1776	In the smallpox epidemic, GEORGE WASHINGTON ordered that the whole army be variolated.
1779	The first book on public health, *System of Medical Policing*, was published in Germany by JOHANN PETER FRANK.
1779	The first cases of Dengue fever were recorded in Batavia, Indonesia and in Cairo.

1781	Start of the worst influenza pandemic in Europe in the eighteenth century. This affected 60% of the population of Rome, 75% of the population of Britain, and spread through the Americas.
1788	DAVID PITCAIRN, a London physician, noted lesions in the heart valves following rheumatic fever, and introduced the term 'rheumatic' in the description of heart disease.
1789	EDWARD DONAVAN born. An Irish pharmacist who prepared and marketed Donovan solution, containing iodides of arsenic and mercury, for application to cutaneous and venereal sores.
1790	LOUIS ODIER, a physician from Geneva, is widely credited as being the first to introduce vaccination, and wrote *A Manual of Practice of Medicine*.
1790	The first accurate clinical description of orchitis associated with mumps was given by ROBERT HAMILTON of Edinburgh.
1791	PIERRE PROSPER BAUME born. A French physician who proposed the theory that a child affected with syphilis will not affect the mother if she has no signs of the disease (Baume law).
1792	English physician WILLIAM WITHERING described the medicinal uses of the plant *Cicuta*, that was used in the treatment of cancer and syphilis.
1793	MICHAEL UNDERWOOD, a London pediatrician, described a form of paralysis following a brief illness in children and published *A Treatise on the Diseases of*

Children, probably the first scientific account of poliomyelitis.

1793 MATTHEW CAREY, an Irish-American physician gave an accurate account of the yellow fever epidemic that struck Philadelphia.

1793 BENJAMIN RUSH wrote *An Account of the Bilious Remitting Yellow Fever, As It Appeared in the City of Philadelphia, in the year 1793*, that killed 5000 in four months.

1795 ALEXANDER GARDEN recognized the association between erysipelas and puerperal fever.

1798 EDWARD JENNER published *An Inquiry into the Causes and Effects of the Variolae Vaccinae*. The first vaccination against smallpox with cowpox pustule liquid was carried out by Jenner, who also gave a description of accelerated secondary local inflammatory response in a smallpox immune patient. By 1801, 100,000 individuals had been vaccinated in England alone.

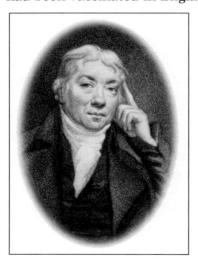

Edward Jenner
(1749–1823)

1798	LOUIS FLORENTINE CALMIEL born. A French physician who found pathological lesions in the brain of patients with general paresis (before the cause of syphilis was known).
1800	The contagiousness of erysipelas was first recognized by American physician, WILLIAM CHARLES WELLS and, in 1810, he described rheumatic nodules in rheumatic fever.
1800	BENJAMIN WATERHOUSE, the first professor of medicine at Harvard, introduced inoculation for smallpox in America and wrote *History of Kinepox*.
1800	Chlorine was used to purify water by Edinburgh surgeon and anatomist, WILLIAM CRUIKSHANK.
1803	LOUIS DANIEL BEAUPERTHUY born. A West Indian pioneer in the field of tropical medicine who noted the causal relationship of mosquitoes to virulent epidemics of yellow fever.
1804	The infectious nature of the saliva of a dog suffering from rabies was proposed by GEORGE GOTTFRIED ZINKE of Jena.
1805	MARY SEACOLE born in Kingston, Jamaica. She was famous for her work in the Crimea among the troops.
1808	Swiss anatomist CARL RUDOLPHI used the term 'echinococcus' for the Taenia group of worms.
1808	British physician CHARLES BADHAM described and named bronchitis. He wrote *Observations on the Inflammatory Affections of the Mucous Membrane of the*

Bronchiae and *Essay on Bronchitis, with Remarks on Pulmonary Abscess* (1814), and distinguished acute and chronic bronchitis from pleuropneumonia and pleurisy.

1808 ROBERT WILLAN used the word lupus to describe cutaneous tuberculosis.

1809 JOHN REID born. A surgeon in Edinburgh who promoted the study of pathology, differentiated between typhoid and typhus fever, and published several treatises on pathology, anatomy and epidemic fevers of Scotland.

1810 GASPARD LAURENT BAYLE, French physician, provided important contributions to an understanding of the pathology of the lung in tuberculosis.

1810 JOHANN VALENTIN VON HILDENBRAND gave a classic description of typhus (Hildenbrand disease).

1810 American physician, NATHAN STRONG gave one of the first and most important descriptions of cerebrospinal meningitis.

1810 JAMES JACKSON JUNIOR, a Boston physician, wrote a treatise on cholera, and described the prolonged expiratory sound in phthisis.

1812 CASIMIR JOSEPH DAVAINE born. A physician from Paris who was an originator of the germ theory of disease before Pasteur, and identified the anthrax bacillus in the blood of animals.

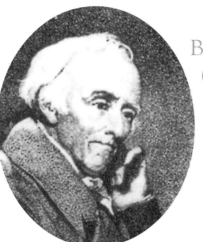

Benjamin Rush
(1745–1813)

Benjamin Waterhouse
(1754–1846)

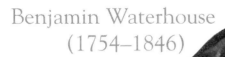

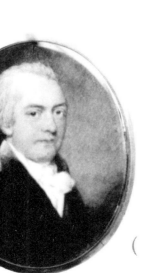

Robert Willan
(1757–1812)

1812	Troop losses due to typhus were a major factor in Napoleon's retreat from Moscow.
1813	One of the first descriptions of herpes genitalis was given by THOMAS BATEMAN, an English surgeon and dermatologist, in *A Practical Synopsis of Cutaneous Diseases*.
1815	LOUIS AUGUSTE FREDERICQ of Belgium born. He described a red line in the gum occurring in the presence of pulmonary tuberculosis (Fredericq sign).
1816	Typhus swept through the British Isles. The Royal Navy remained free of typhus by adopting the recommendations of JAMES LIND, that sailors should be stripped, scrubbed, shaved and issued with clean clothes.
1816	JOHN HASLAM of London examined the brains of the insane at autopsy and recorded changes in the brain due to syphilis.
1818	GEORGE BALLINGALL, professor of military surgery from Edinburgh, described Madura foot, Ballingall disease, and also clarified the difference between bacillary dysentery and amebic dysentery in 1808.
1819	RENE LAENNEC invented the stethoscope. This, and auscultation, allowed him to follow the developmental effects of tuberculosis.
1820	English physician, JAMES CARSON performed open pneumothorax as treatment for pulmonary tuberculosis, and suggested that lungs collapsed if the negative pressure was compromised.

Dates in Infectious Diseases

1823 ARISTIDE VERNEUIL born. A French surgeon who described the syphilitic involvement of the bursae (Verneuil disease), and introduced iodoform as treatment for the common cold.

1824 NATHAN SMITH, a surgeon from Connecticut, described the contagious nature of typhoid in his treatise, *A Practical Essay on Typhus Fever*.

1825 JEAN BAPTISTE EMIL VIDAL born. A French dermatologist who was responsible for the introduction of an efficient sewage system for Paris. He published papers on the use of mercury in syphilis and chaulmoogra oil in leprosy, treatment of gonorrhea, inoculability of impetigo, herpes, ecthyma, mycosis fungoides, lupus erythematosus, tuberculosis, and facial erysipelas. He was successful in treatment of herpes labialis, herpes praeputialis and ecthyma, but not with herpes zona or eczema.

1826 The first clinical description of diphtheria, and its name, was given by PIERRE BRETONNEAU of France. He distinguished it from other forms of pharyngitis, and gave a classic description of typhoid.

1828 ULYSSES TRELAT born. A French surgeon who described small yellowish spots near tuberculous ulcers of the mouth (Trelat sign).

1828 SIR BENJAMIN COLLINS BRODIE described an abscess of long bones due to *Staphylococcus aureus* (Brodie abscess).

1829 JEAN LUGOL, a French pathologist, developed Lugol iodine, 5% iodine and 10% potassium iodide, as a treatment for tuberculosis. The solution was found to have little effect in treating tuberculosis but was later used in thyrotoxicosis.

1829 PIERRE CHARLES LOUIS, a Paris physician, introduced the term 'fievre typhoide' for typhoid fever. He was also a leading authority on tuberculosis.

1829 An influenza epidemic started in Asia and spread to Russia in 1830 and Indonesia by 1831, reaching the USA by November.

1830 London physician, JOHN HUXMAN, published *Observations on Fever*.

1830 THOMAS SOUTHWOOD SMITH, an English Unitarian minister, observed epidemics of fever at the London Fever Hospital, and published *A Treatise on Fever*.

1831 The first suggestion that herpes zoster (caused by the varicella zoster virus) was spread along a nerve was made by RICHARD BRIGHT of Guy's Hospital, London.

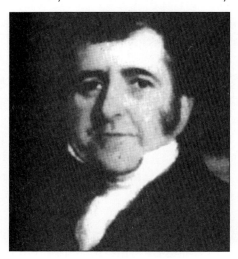

Richard Bright
(1789–1858)

1831	HENRY VANDYKE CARTER born. A physician in the Indian Medical Service who described Madura foot, scrotal elephantiasis and several other diseases.
1831	Potassium iodide was used as a treatment for secondary syphilis by ROBERT WILLIAMS of St Thomas' Hospital, London.
1831	England's first case of cholera, part of the second pandemic in Europe that lasted from 1829 to 1851.
1832	JEAN BAPTISTE BOUILLAUD, a French physician, correlated carditis with acute rheumatic fever (Bouillaud syndrome), described acute rheumatic polyarthritis, and related the occurrence of endocarditis to acute rheumatism.
1832	JEAN ALFRED FOURNIER of Paris born. He made important contributions to the study of syphilis, and gave his name to fulminating gangrene of the scrotum and perineum in diabetic patients.
1832	JOHN PARKIN born. An English surgeon who described the use of charcoal filters to purify water and therefore prevent the spread of cholera.
1832	DANIEL DRAKE of Cincinnati wrote *A Practical Treatise on the History, Prevention, and Treatment of Epidemic Cholera, Designed both for the Professional and the People*. Records showed 50% mortality in Montreal and Quebec, 5000 deaths in New Orleans and 3000 deaths in New York.
1832	Intravenous saline was first used as treatment for circulatory collapse following cholera by THOMAS AITCHISON LATTA.

1834	Tuberculosis spondylitis of the cervical vertebrae (Rust disease) was described by German surgeon, JOHANN NEPOMAK RUST.
1835	Irish surgeon, ABRAHAM COLLES wrote a treatise on syphilis, *Practical Observation on the Venereal Disease*, in which he referred to immunity acquired to syphilis by a healthy mother in bearing a syphilitic child (Colles law).
1835	PASTEUR developed the first antirabies treatment, using the spinal cord of an infected rabbit.
1835	The fungal cause of muscardine disease of the silkworm (silkworm disease) was discovered by Italian, AGOSTINO BASSI, this was considered to be the first proof for pathogenesis of germs.
1837	ARMAND TROUSSEAU of France received the prize of the Academy of Medicine for his treatise on laryngeal phthisis.

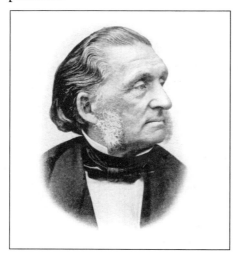

Armand Trousseau
(1801–1867)

1837	American physician, WILLIAM WOOD GERHARD gave an early, clear clinicopathological description of typhoid, and made an accurate study of tuberculous meningitis (1834).
1837	JOHANN LUCAS SCHÖNLEIN, a German professor, introduced the terms hemophilia and tuberculosis, and described peliosis rheumatica (Schönlein disease or purpura rheumatica).
1838	PHILLIPE RICORD, an American pioneer in venereology, published his work on the different etiology of syphilis and gonorrhea, and described the three stages of syphilis.
1838	Curare was first used in medical practice to relax the muscles in rabies.
1839	GEORG DIEULAFOY born. A French professor who described gastric ulceration as a complication of pneumonia (Dieulafoy disease), and worked on Bright disease, typhoid and appendicitis.
1840	GIUSEPPE PROFETA born. A Sicilian physician who proposed the law (Profeta law) that an apparent healthy infant will not be affected by its syphilitic mother.
1840	A clear differentiation between typhus and typhoid fever was made by ALEXANDER PATRICK STEWART.
1840	The causative organism of cholera, *Vibrio cholerae*, was discovered by Italian professor FILIPPO PACINI.

1840	*Streptobacillus monoliformis* was shown as the cause of rat bite fever by a physician in the Indian Medical Service, HENRY VANDYKE CARTER, 47 years after the first report was made by WHITMAN WILCOX.
1840	VLADIMIR KERNIG born. A Russian neurologist who described how flexion of the thigh at the hip and extension of the leg causes pain and spasm in the hamstrings, in cases of meningitis.
1840	JACOB VON HEINE, a German orthopedist, gave one of the first descriptions of 'infantile spinal paralysis' or poliomyelitis. In the same year he wrote of the nature of germs: '[they are] animate, indeed endowed with individual life.'
1842	WILLIAM FARR suggested that infection was the result of 'multiplying ferments' generated during decomposition of living material.
1843	OLIVER WENDELL HOLMES gave a paper to the Boston Society for Medical Improvement on 'The Contagiousness of Puerperal Fever' saying 'it would seem incredible that any should be found too prejudiced or indolent to accept the solemn truth knelled into their ears by the funeral bells from both sides of the ocean... the plain conclusion that the physician and the disease enter hand in hand, into the chamber of the unsuspecting patient.'
1843	The presence of albumin in the urine (albuminuria) of mothers with puerperal convulsions, was observed by JOHN CHARLES LEVER of Guy's Hospital in London.

1844	WILLIAM HENDERSON, a Scottish physician, was one of the first to differentiate typhus from relapsing fever, and wrote a treatise on the skin disease, molluscum contagiosum.
1845	ELIE METCHNIKOFF born. An immunologist and embryologist from the Ukraine who, while director of the Pasteur Institute in Paris, discovered the phagocytic function of white blood cells and demonstrated their role in combating bacterial invasion. He shared the Nobel Prize in 1908 with Paul Ehrlich, for their contributions to immunity and serum therapy.
1845	JOHN ELLIOT WOODBRIDGE born. An American physician who used an intestinal antiseptic containing calomel (Woodbridge treatment) in the treatment of typhoid.
1846	A term for typhoid, enteric fever, was coined by CHARLES RITCHIE of England.
1846	HORACE GREEN of Vermont wrote on chronic laryngitis and bronchitis in *Treatise on the Diseases of the Air Passages*.
1846	Danish physician, PETER LUDWIG PANUM described the epidemiology of measles and gave the first scientific explanation and description of how a disease spreads from person to person and from place to place.
1847	The term scleroderma was coined by GINTRAC, after an early attempt to differentiate scleroderma from leprosy and other skin diseases was made by Italian physician, CARLO CURZIO.

1847	PAUL LANGERHANS born. He researched and wrote on leprosy and the spread of tuberculosis. His inaugural dissertation was *Communication on the Microscopic Anatomy of the Pancreas*. Langerhans cells produce the immune response in contact dermatitis and the antigenic response through the lymphatic system.
1847	Russian pediatrician, NILS FEODOROVITCH FILATOV born. He described the characteristic features of lymphadenopathy and fever seen in infectious mononucleosis (glandular fever).
1847	IGNAZ SEMMELWEISS, a Hungarian obstetrician, demonstrated that mortality due to puerperal fever could be reduced from 18% to less than 2% if doctors washed their hands.
1848	EDWARD LIVINGSTON TRUDEAU born. A New York physician who pioneered fresh air therapy for tuberculosis.
1848	DANIEL CORNELIUS DANIELSSEN and CARL WILHELM BOECK wrote the first treatise on leprosy. Danielssen disease is a form of anesthetic polyneuritis in leprosy.
1848	JOSEPH CLARK NOTT of Mobile suggested that the mosquito might carry yellow fever but he had no hard evidence.
1850	The absence or multiple abscesses in the thymus, in cases of congenital syphilis (Dubois disease), was described by PAUL DUBOIS of Paris.
1850	HANS BÜCHNER born. A German bacteriologist who carried out pioneering work on proteins in the blood (gammaglobulins) that combine with invading organisms and protect against infections.

Dates in Infectious Diseases

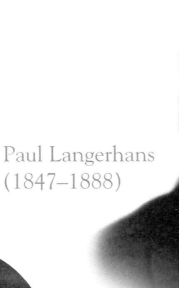

Paul Langerhans
(1847–1888)

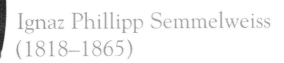

Ignaz Phillipp Semmelweiss
(1818–1865)

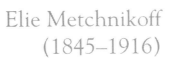

Elie Metchnikoff
(1845–1916)

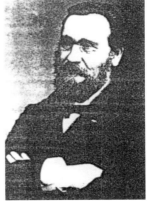

1851	GEORGE THOMPSON ELLIOT born. An American dermatologist who described the Elliot sign of induration at the periphery of certain syphilitic skin lesions.
1851	WALTER REED born in Belroi, Virginia. In 1900 he was appointed president of a board to study infectious diseases in Cuba, particularly yellow fever. Reed was buried in Arlington National Cemetery, where an inscription reads: 'He gave to man control over that dreadful scourge, yellow fever.'
1851	*Schistosoma*, the bilharzia parasite, was discovered by THEODOR MAXIMILIAN BILHARZ, a German professor in Cairo.
1852	The shallow glass dish for use in culturing bacteria (Petri dish) was designed by German bacteriologist, RICHARD JULIUS PETRI.
1852	SHIBASABURO KITASATO born. A Japanese bacteriologist who isolated the causative organism of bubonic plague, *Pasteurella pestis* (1894), independently of ALEXANDRE YERSIN. In 1890, with EMIL VON BEHRING, he performed the first successful clinical test of diphtheria antitoxin and proposed the word 'alexin' for the substance which was later renamed 'complement'.
1853	JULES COMBY born. A French pediatrician who described the whitish-yellow patches seen in inflamed buccal mucosa before the onset of Koplik spots in measles (Comby sign).
1854	FRIEDRICH ADOLF NEELSEN born. A German

pathologist who developed the acid-fast method of staining mycobacteria.

1854 German physician, FRIEDRICH VON BÄRENSPRUNG described Bärensprung disease, an acute or chronic fungal and contagious skin infection caused by *Tinea cruris*.

1854 JOHN SNOW removed the pump handle from the Broad Street drinking water pump in London and stopped the spread of cholera. Snow concluded that cholera was spread by germs in the water.

1855 Scottish surgeon, SIR JAMES RONALD MARTIN published a treatise on tropical diseases, *Influence of Tropical Climates on European Constitutions*.

1857 LOUIS PASTEUR provided evidence that organisms invisible to the naked eye were responsible for fermentation. He then proved that fermentation and putrefaction occur after exposure to air.

1858 Curare was first used in medical practice to relax the muscles in tetanus.

1858 ERNST TAVEL born. A Swiss surgeon from Bern who prepared one of the first antistreptococcal sera (Tavel serum).

1859 THEOBALD SMITH born. An American bacteriologist who showed that a tick (the first insect vector discovered) caused Texas cattle fever, distinguished human and bovine tuberculosis, and made important contributions to vaccine development.

1860	The first complete life history and morphology of *Echinococcus* was provided by German zoologist, KARL GEORG LEUCKART.
1861	Interstitial keratitis, deafness, and pegged incisor teeth in congenital syphilis (Hutchinson triad) were described by JONATHAN HUTCHINSON.
1861	DIMITRI ROMANOVSKY born. A Russian physician who devised Romanovsky stain (eosin and methylene blue stain for studying blood films), which he used to demonstrate that malarial parasites were damaged during treatment with quinine.
1861	KARL HERXHEIMER born. A German dermatologist who described chronic atrophic acrodermatitis and acute exacerbation of syphilitic lesions within 6-10 hours of the initiation of treatment (Herxheimer reaction).
1861	Infection of the sweat gland accompanied by collection of fluid or pus (hydroadentitis) was first described by ERNEST BAZIN of France.
1861	ALFRED MACCONKEY born. An English bacteriologist who invented MacConkey agar, used for the culture of bacteria, and consisting of a mixture of malachite green, bile, dextrose and meat extract.
1862	*A Treatise on the Continued Fevers of Great Britain* was written by London physician, CHARLES MURCHISON.
1863	Leptospirosis (Weil disease) was described by JEFFREY ALLEN MARSTON after ADOLF WEIL had published four cases of infectious jaundice with hemorrhage.

Dates in Infectious Diseases

1863   Louis Pasteur developed pasteurization. He distinguished aerobic and anaerobic organisms and suggested that infectious diseases were caused by living organisms called 'germs.'

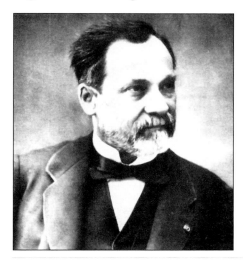

Louis Pasteur (1822–1895)

1864   The Contagious Diseases Act, an act of Parliament designed to combat the spread of venereal diseases, was passed in England.

1864   The endemic status of bilharziasis in South Africa was shown by John Harley.

1864   Frederick George Novy born. A professor of bacteriology in Michigan, who identified the causative organism of American relapsing fever, the body louse (*Pediculus humanis corporis*).

1864   Robert Koch of Germany devised a staining and fixing method for bacteria, developing a method of producing pure cultures which facilitated the isolation of the genus, *Bacillus anthracis*, followed by its growth in culture in 1876.

1865   The contagiousness of tuberculosis was demonstrated by French surgeon, JEAN-ANTOINE VILLEMIN. He showed that it could be passed from humans to cattle and from cattle to rabbits. He postulated a specific microorganism as the cause.

1865   JOSEPH LISTER conducted the first operation using antiseptic techniques. He first observed the antibacterial properties of *Penicillium* when he used a crude preparation to treat an infected wound. The causative gram positive bacterium of meningitis, lymphadenopathy and pyrexia found in immunosuppressed patients, *Listeria monocytogenes*, is named in his honor.

1866   Carbolic acid was used as a disinfectant during the cholera epidemic in London, and was also employed for the deodorization of sewage. JOSEPH LISTER devised a hand-driven carbolic acid spray for disinfection during surgery. The spray was later steam-driven and remained in use for the next two decades.

1866   ANTON GHON born. He was an Austrian pathologist who described a calcified area of the lung (Ghon focus), shown on chest X-ray, and due to healed primary tuberculosis.

1866   Tabetic gastric crisis with paroxysms of severe abdominal pain in patients with tabetic syphilis were described by GEORGES DELMARRE of Paris.

1867   LOUIS PASTEUR demonstrated that germs caused disease. He developed pasteurization, a method of partial heat sterilization at 55 to 60°C to prevent fermentation by microorganisms or vinegar formation

Lister's carbolic acid spray

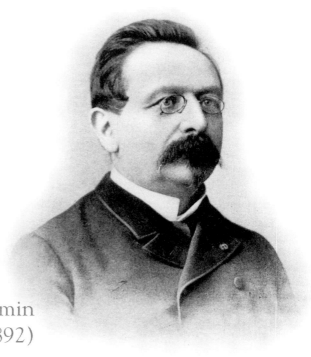

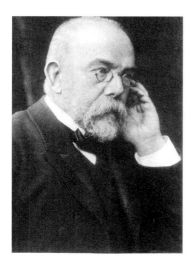

Heinrich Hermann
Robert Koch
(1843–1910)

Jean-Antoine Villemin
(1827–1892)

in wine. He went on to develop vaccines for chicken cholera, anthrax and rabies.

1868   The causative spirochete of relapsing fever transmitted by the human louse (*Borrelia obermeyeri*) was discovered by German physician, OTTO OBERMEYER.

1868   AUGUSTE CHAUVEAU of Paris was the first to demonstrate experimentally in animals that swallowing tubercular matter led to ulceration in the intestines (intestinal tuberculosis).

1868   KARL WUNDERLICH published *On the Temperature in Disease*.

1869   JOSEPH LISTER introduced catgut treated with carbolic acid to promote asepsis.

1870   ALEXEI P. FEDCHENKO elucidated the life-cycle of *Dracunculus medinensis* and identified the cyclops as its intermediate host.

1870   JEAN-MARTIN CHARCOT and A. JOFFROY noted microscopic changes in the anterior horn cells of the spinal cord in polio victims.

1871   HOWARD TAYLOR RICKETTS born. A microbiologist from the United States who showed that the causative agent of Rocky Mountain spotted fever was transmitted by ticks, and who researched the causative organism of Mexican typhus fever.

1871   A bacterial filter made of porous clay to separate anthrax bacteria from the medium was made by TIEGEL.

Dates in Infectious Diseases

1873   William Budd published *Typhoid Fever: Its Nature, Mode of Spreading and Prevention*. He proposed excreta as a source of typhoid.

1873   Hansen bacillus, *Mycobacterium leprae*, the causative organism of leprosy, was discovered by Norwegian bacteriologist, Gerhard Hansen.

1873   Georges Dreyer born. An English pathologist who introduced a modified form of the Widal test for diagnosis of typhoid and paratyphoid (Dreyer test).

1873   German bacteriologist, Theodor Klebs pointed out the tuberculous cavities in the lungs as a source of intestinal tuberculosis.

1874   Austin Flint wrote on 'the logical proof of the contagiousness and non-contagiousness of diseases.' This contained the first mention of bacteria in American scientific literature.

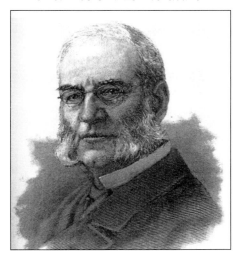

Austin Flint
(1812–1886)

1874	FREDERICK PARKER GAY born. An American pathologist who studied the cell count in cerebrospinal fluid in poliomyelitis.
1874	GEORGES HAYEM of Paris described chronic interstitial hepatitis, gave the first accurate account of blood platelets, and identified the early stage of red cells during regeneration.
1876	C.S. KRISHNASWAMI born. An Indian physician who described the Whitmore bacillus (the causative organism of melidiosis), with ALFRED WHITMORE.
1876	The first molars in congenital syphilis (Moon molars), were described by a dental surgeon from Guy's Hospital, London, HENRY MOON.
1876	JUSTIN LUCAS-CHAMPIONNIERE of Paris introduced the Listerian system of antiseptic surgery into France and described chronic pseudomembranous bronchitis (Lucas-Championniere disease).
1876	ROBERT KOCH demonstrated the cause of anthrax in horses by isolating anthrax bacilli and showing their ability to cause disease and their capacity to form spores. Koch proved that specific organisms could cause specific diseases and produced four postulates to confirm causal links between an organism (parasite) and a disease. Koch also developed culture techniques for bacteria, steam sterilization, and discovered the tubercle bacillus was the cause of clinical tuberculosis.
1876	The intestinal parasitic roundworm that causes diarrhea (*Strongyloides stercoralis*) was described by LOUIS NORMAND in Cochin, China.

Dates in Infectious Diseases

1877   WALTER BUTLER CHEADLE proved that rickets and scurvy (Cheadle disease) were two different diseases.

1877   Juvenile paresis was associated with congenital syphilis by SIR THOMAS CLOUSTON from Orkney, a superintendent at the Royal Morningside Asylum.

1877   Austrian neurologist, JULIUS WAGNER-JAUREGG, introduced shock therapy for syphilis, following the introduction of fever therapy for syphilis and other diseases.

1878   The fungus *Actinomyces israelii* was discovered by German urologist JAMES ADOLPH ISRAEL.

1878   Austrian dermatologist, GOTTFRIED RITTER VON RIETTSHAIM described dermatitis exfoliativa neonatorum (Ritter disease), now known to be caused by a staphylococcal infection (scalded skin syndrome).

1878   Scrub typhus (originally known as Shima-mushi or island insect disease) was first observed in Japan.

1878   A yellow fever epidemic struck more than 100 towns in the USA, killing at least 20,000 people.

1878   CARLOS FINLAY of Cuba proposed that yellow fever was caused by a virus that was vectored by mosquitoes.

1878   ERNEST LOWENSTEIN born. A Viennese pathologist who (with Danish bacteriologist, ORLA JENSEN) prepared the Lowenstein–Jensen medium, used to culture *Mycobacterium tuberculosis*.

1878 THEODOR KLEBS successfully transmitted syphilis to monkeys. He also studied malaria, hemorrhagic pancreatitis, and noted that bacteria cause septicemia. A genus of bacteria, *Klebsiella*, are named after him, the best known of which, *K. pneumoniae*, is a cause of respiratory tract infections such as pneumonia.

1878 HANS ZINSSER born. An American bacteriologist who worked on allergy, virus size, typhus and causes of rheumatic fever, differentiated between epidemics from endemic ricketssial typhus, and wrote *Rats, Lice and History* (1934) on typhus fever.

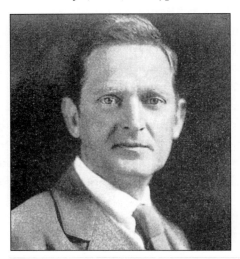

Hans Zinsser (1878–1940)

1879 A paralytic form of rabies was produced by VICTOR GALTIER of Paris.

1879 French physician, JULES MARIE PARROT described the Parrot nodes, nodules in the skulls of infants with congenital syphilis, and the Parrot sign of dilatation of the pupils induced by pinching the skin of the neck of patients with meningitis.

1879   PATRICK MANSON identified the *Anopheles* mosquito as a vector for filariasis and proposed the extracorporeal life cycle for the parasite.

1879   ALBERT LUDWIG NEISSER, a German bacteriologist, discovered the gonorrhea bacterium (*Neisseria gonorrhoeae*). He gave a complete review of the hydatid disease in his treatise *Die Echinococcenkrankheit* (1877).

1879   Psittacosis (parrot fever) was first described by JACOB RITTER in Switzerland, and the sources of many outbreaks were traced to consignments of diseased parrots.

1880   The causative organism of enteric fever (typhoid), *Salmonella typhi*, was discovered by CARL JOSEPH EBERTH, professor of pathology at Halle.

1880   SIR JAMES KINGSTON FOWLER, London physician, noted the association between throat infections and acute rheumatism. He later proposed that pulmonary tuberculosis spread from the apex of the dorsal lobe along the greater fissure to the periphery.

1880   French parasitologist, CHARLES LOUIS LAVERAN studied malaria in Algiers and discovered the causative organism, a protozoan parasite, *Plasmodium*.

1881   The protective effect of inoculating small doses of anthrax bacilli in animals which paved the way for active immunization was explained by LOUIS PASTEUR. He was also credited with the first vaccinations against fowl cholera, sheep anthrax, swine erysipelas, and rabies in dogs and humans.

1881	CARLOS FINLAY of Havana, Cuba presented a paper, *The Mosquito Hypothetically Considered as the Agent of Transmission of Yellow Fever*, suggesting a 'transportable substance, which may be an amorphous virus, a vegetable or animal germ, a bacterium, etc.'
1881	Italian physician, LUIGI CONCATO described polyserositis due to tuberculosis.
1881	Scottish surgeon, ALEXANDER OGSTON discovered *Staphylococcus* bacteria and described the imaginary line (Ogston line) used in surgery that extends from a tubercle of the femur to the intercondylar notch.
1882	ARTHUR JAMES EWINS born. An English chemist who isolated the neurotransmitter acetylcholine, and whose work led to the development of the antibiotic, sulfapyridine, which was the first successful treatment for gonorrhea.
1882	HEINRICH IRANAEUS QUINCKE of Germany gave an account of angioneurotic edema and distinguished between *Entamoeba histolytica* and *Entamoeba coli*.
1882	German bacteriologist, ROBERT KOCH, identified the tubercle bacillus, the first bacteria attributed to a human disease. A year later he identified the cholera bacterium.
1882	CARL FRIEDLÄNDER of Germany discovered and isolated the Friedländer bacillus (*Klebsiella pneumoniae*) from a series of patients with pneumonia caused by this Gram-negative bacillus.

Dates in Infectious Diseases

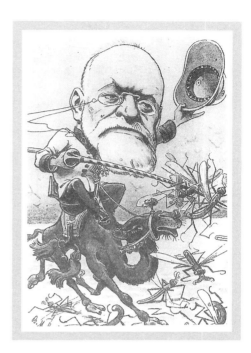

Charles Louis Alphonse Laveran (1845–1922)

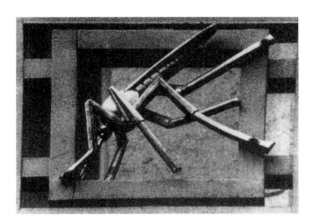

Sculpture of the Anopheles mosquito by Allan Gairdner Wyon used to decorate the London School of Hygiene and Tropical Medicine

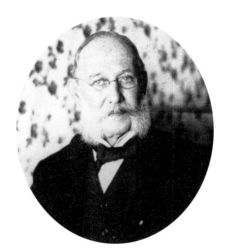

Carlos Juan Finlay (1833–1915)

1882 ERNST VICTOR VON LEYDEN of Germany worked on tabes and poliomyelitis, established sanatoria for treatment of tuberculosis, was the first to describe fatty infiltration of the heart, gave a concise account of heart disease and described the crystalline sputum in asthmatics.

1883 American physician, ALBERT FREEMAN AFRICANUS KING, was one of the first to associate transmission of malaria with the mosquito.

1884 The Gram stain for classifying bacteria was developed by HANS CHRISTIAN GRAM of Denmark, while working on methods for double-staining kidney sections.

1884 JOHN ELMER WEEKS of New York, an ophthalmologist, discovered the bacillus (Koch-Weeks bacillus, *Haemophilus aegyptius*) of epidemic mucopurulent bilateral conjunctivitis (pink disease).

1884 The infectious nature of herpes zoster was first recognized by French physician, LOUIS LANDOUZY.

1884 GEORG THEODOR GAFFKY, a German bacteriologist from Hannover, obtained a pure culture of *Salmonella typhi* and demonstrated it caused typhoid.

1884 JULIUS FRIEDRICH ROSENBACH of Germany introduced the name *Streptococcus* for the cocci found in chains, and differentiated between staphylococci and streptococci.

1884 CHARLES CHAMBERLAND of France devised a new bacterial filtering device which was later modified by Louis Pasteur.

Dates in Infectious Diseases

1884   Karl Weigert of Germany devised some of the earliest and best staining methods for studying bacteria and histological tissues.

1884   Theodor Klebs and Friedrich Löffler discovered the diphtheria bacillus (*Corynebacterium diphtheriae*), also known as the Klebs–Löffler bacillus.

1885   The bacterium, *Escherichia coli*, was named after the German bacteriologist Theodor Escherich, who gave the first account of the bacillus infection in children.

1885   *Salmonella* was named after Daniel Elmer Salmon of Cornell University, who isolated American hog cholera bacillus while working with Theobald Smith at the US Bureau of Animal Industry.

1885   Bacteria were implicated in rheumatic fever by Sir William Osler, in his paper *Malignant Endocarditis*.

1885   J. Ferran, a Spanish bacteriologist, made the first attempt at immunization against cholera on a large scale, during an outbreak of the disease in Spain.

1885   Ettore Marchiafava of Italy described malarial parasites in red blood cells as 'hemocytozoa' and gave a description of *Plasmodium* (1880).

1885   Pasteur's rabies vaccine, developed from the stored infected brains of animals, was used to treat a young boy who had been bitten by a rabid dog. He used the Latin word, 'vacca' meaning cow for his new 'vaccine.'

1886   Elizabeth Kenny born. A pioneer of nursing in Australia who established clinics for providing physical therapy to polio victims in Britain and America.

1886	Weil's disease (caused by *Leptospira*) first described.
1886	GEORGE MILLER STERNBERG published *Disinfection and Individual Prophylaxis against Infectious Diseases*.
1886	German physician, ALBERT FRAENKEL, discovered *Diplococcus pneumoniae* (*Streptococcus pneumoniae*), commonly called pneumococcus.
1887	The infectious nature of acute anterior poliomyelitis was clinically described by OSCAR MEDIN after studying a large breakout of this disease in Sweden.
1887	ANTON WEICHELSBAUM of Austria isolated meningococcus, or *Diplococcus intercellularis meningitides*, from the cerebrospinal fluid of patients with meningitis.
1887	The bacterium in the spleen of patients dying from Mediterranean fever (*Brucellosis*) was isolated by SIR DAVID BRUCE who named it *Mirococcus melitensis*.
1887	Mercury injections were introduced as a treatment for syphilis by P. HEPP of Germany, but abandoned due to toxicity.
1888	An important landmark in the study of bacterial food poisoning was the discovery of *Salmonella enteritidis* as a cause of meat poisoning by Austrian physician GUSTAV GAERTNER during an outbreak at Frankenhausen.
1888	CARLO FORLANINI of Italy established induction of pneumothorax as a regular treatment for pulmonary tuberculosis.

Dates in Infectious Diseases

1888   Sir Robert William Philip, Scottish pioneer in the study and control of tuberculosis, established the first tuberculosis dispensary in the world in Edinburgh.

1888   French bacteriologist André Chantemmesse isolated the dysentery bacillus.

1888   Symptoms of fever, vomiting, irritability and headache in cerebrospinal fever were described by Sir William Richard Gowers, the British neurologist. In 1902 he introduced the term 'abiotrophy' to focus attention on diseases not caused by infection.

1889   A classic description of infectious mononucleosis (Pfeiffer disease) as 'Drüsenfieber' was given by Emil Pfeiffer of Germany.

1889   Augusto Ducrey, an Italian dermatologist, described the sexually transmitted causative organism of chancroid which was later named *Haemophilis ducreyi* in his honor.

1889   Diphtheria was shown to be due to the toxin and not the bacterium, by French bacteriologists, Pierre Roux and Alexander Emile Jean Yersin, and, in 1894, Roux discovered the cure for diphtheria using serum from immunized horses.

1889   Bismuth was suggested as a treatment for syphilis by Paris physician, Felix Balzar.

1889   Start of the so-called Russian flu epidemic. This worldwide epidemic began in Central Asia, spread north to Russia, east to China, west to Europe, then hit North America, parts of Africa and Pacific Rim countries. It is estimated that three-quarters of a million people were killed.

1890 FRIEDRICH LÖFFLER noted structures in bacteria (flagella) which enabled motility and in collaboration with PAUL FROSCH in 1897 showed that foot and mouth disease in animals was caused by a filterable agent.

1890 WILLIAM HALSTEAD invented rubber gloves for use in surgery.

1890 ANGELO MAFFUCCI of Italy, a pioneer in the study of tuberculosis, isolated the avian tubercle bacillus (*B. gallinaceous*), and described Maffucci syndrome (endochondromatosis with cutaneous hemangioma).

1890 The intestinal disease amebic dysentery was studied and named by WILLIAM COUNCILMAN of Harvard University.

1890 EMIL VON BEHRING and SHIBASABURO KITASATO immunized animals against diphtheria and tetanus using antibodies from blood of previously infected animals. They wrote: 'Blood serum which has developed immunity against diphtheria or tetanus exerts an antitoxic effect on the toxin in the infected organism.'

1891 Strümpell disease (polioencephalomyelitis) was described by a German neurologist, ERNST VON STRÜMPELL from Leipzig.

1891 A.C. ABBOTT at Johns Hopkins Hospital found a strain of *Staphylococcus aureus* which could withstand exposure to mercuric chloride.

William Stewart Halsted
(1852–1922)

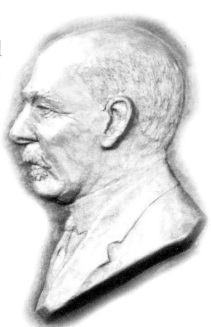

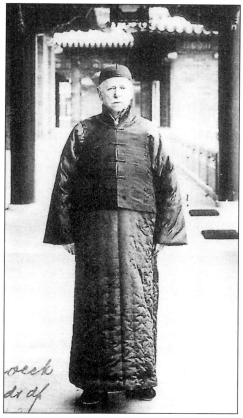

William Thomas
Councilman
(1854–1933)

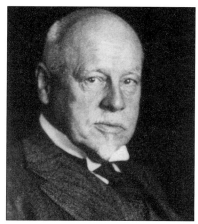

William Henry
Welch
(1850–1934)

1891	American pathologist, WILLIAM HENRY WELCH, studied diphtheria toxin and discovered the anaerobic organism isolated from patients with gas gangrene, *Clostridium welchii*.
1892	Plague epidemics lasting four years occurred in China and India.
1892	The occurrence of chickenpox following exposure to cases of herpes lesions was observed by JANOS VON B¢KAY of Germany.
1892	A reddish eruption on the soft palate in cases of rubella (Forchheimer sign) was first described by American physician, FREDERICK FORCHHEIMER.
1892	The first work on ringworm of the hands and feet was published by DJELALEDDIN-MOUKHTAR, a physician to the Ottoman army.
1892	The first description of the Döderlein bacillus in vaginal secretions in relation to puerperal fever was given by German gynecologist, ALBERT DÖDERLEIN.
1892	RICHARD PFEIFFER, a Polish bacteriologist discovered *Haemophilus influenzae*, and later demonstrated bacteriolysis which provided the first scientific evidence for the presence of antibodies.
1892	The causative organism of mycosis fungoides was discovered in Buenos Aires, Argentina, by ALEJANDRO POSADAS and later named 'coccidioides imitis.'
1892	Leprosy was endemic in Louisiana, mostly among whites. The state sent patients to a smallpox hospital

in New Orleans. In 1921, the Federal Government annexed the property and patients and it became the only US Public Health Service Hospital devoted exclusively to leprosy.

1892 Tobacco mosaic disease was investigated by Russian botanist DMITRI ISOFOVITCH, the first demonstration of a filterable virus.

1892 EMIL VON BEHRING published *History of Diphtheria* and *Review on the Etiological Therapy of Infectious Diseases*.

1893 The sixth cholera pandemic erupted in the Middle East, Russia, and other parts of Europe. This came at a time when immigration into New York was high. Jewish immigrants were targeted and sent to North Brother Island, downwind of the garbage dump on Riker's Island.

1893 Russian physician, WALDEMAR HAFFKINE, pioneered inoculation against cholera in India and conducted an antiplague vaccination program using live vaccine in the village of Mulkowal, accidentally killing 19 people with tetanus.

1893 ERICH URBACH born. A Czech biochemist, dermatologist and expert in venereal disease, who worked on the interaction of cutaneous disease with allergy and diet.

1894 The plague bacillus, *Pasteurella pestis* (or *Yersinia pestis*) was isolated from humans independently by Swiss bacteriologist ALEXANDER YERSIN and SHIBASABURO KITASATO.

1894	The last major infestation of plague (over a million died) arose in China and Hong Kong.
1894	EDWARD LIVINGSTON TRUDEAU founded the Trudeau Sanatorium for patients with tuberculosis, at a cottage called Little Red, housing two 'frail, ill-clad factory girls.' He employed open-air treatment of the disease and organized the first laboratory for the study of tuberculosis.
1894	JEAN DANYSZ, Polish pathologist, studied rat plague, and described a decrease in antitoxin neutralizing capacity when toxin is added incrementally rather than all at once (Danysz phenomenon).
1894	Nasher fever, involving mucous membrane of the upper respiratory tract with toxic symptoms, occurring mainly in India, was described by FERNANDEZ at the Indian Medical Congress.
1894	SIR PATRICK MANSON, the father of tropical medicine and founder of the London School of Tropical Medicine (1899), described the relationship of malaria to mosquito bites and proposed the extracorporeal lifecycle for the malarial parasite. His *Tropical Diseases* was published in 1898, and he described the skin disease tinea nigra (caused by *Cladosporium mansoni*).
1895	American, GEORGE MARTIN KOBER, pointed out that flies are carriers of typhoid fever. He was a pioneer in industrial hygiene in America.
1895	SIR LIONEL WHITBY from the University of Cambridge proved the efficacy of sulfapyridine in the treatment of pneumococcal pneumonia.

Dates in Infectious Diseases

1895 Italian bacteriologist, ACHILLE SCLAVO, developed an antiserum for anthrax.

1895 The Bacille Calmette–Guérin vaccine (BCG) for tuberculosis was developed by the founder of the Pasteur Institute in Lille, France, LEON CHARLES ALBERT CALMETTE (with ALPHONSE GUÉRIN).

1895 WILHELM KONRAD RÖNTGEN discovered X-rays.

1895 A subacute form of infection of the nervous system caused by the organism *Cryptococcus neoformans* was described by Berlin dermatologist, ABRAHAM BUSCHKE.

1895 Circulatory collapse in cerebrospinal meningitis (Waterhouse-Friderichsen syndrome) was described by ARTHUR FRANCIS VOELCKER.

1896 Rocky Mountain spotted fever was found in the Montana and Idaho districts of America and was first described by EDWARD ERNEST MAXEY.

1896 The Babinski syndrome, associated with cardioaortic syphilis and neurosyphilis, was described by JULES FRANÇOIS BABINSKI.

1896 JOHANN OTTO HEUBNER of Germany isolated meningococci from cerebrospinal fluid, described syphilitic endarteritis of cerebral vessels and the infantile form of idiopathic steatorrhoea.

1896 The etiological agent of botulism, *Clostridium*, was isolated by Belgian bacteriologist, ÉMILE VAN ERMENGEN, during investigations into a small outbreak in Ellezeles, Belgium.

1896	The great American physician, WILLIAM OSLER, addressed the American Medical Association on 'The Study of the Fevers of the South'. It commenced, 'Humanity has but three great enemies: fever, famine and war; of these by far the greatest, by far the most terrible, is fever.'
1896	LEOPOLD FREUND first observed the effect of X-rays on the skin in the treatment of ringworm infection.
1896	The Gram-negative bacterium, Morax-Axenfeld bacillus, was described as a cause of angular conjunctivitis in man by Swiss ophthalmologist in Paris, VICTOR MORAX.
1896	JOHN BROWN BUIST of Edinburgh described the elementary body in the skin lesions seen in smallpox and vaccinia (Buist-Paschen) that appear as minute particles in stained smears of vaccinial lesions.
1896	LEE FOSHAY born. An American bacteriologist who devised a skin test for the diagnosis of tularemia, and prepared a serum for its treatment.
1897	A genus of flea (*Xenopsylla cheopis*) was shown to be a plague vector by Masanori Ogata. The mode of transmission of plague was clarified by P.L. SIMOND.
1897	KIYOSHI SHIGA of Japan discovered the bacillus of dysentery (*Shigella shigae*).
1897	British Nobel laureate RONALD ROSS discovered the life cycle of the avian parasite responsible for the transmission of malaria to birds by bites from infected mosquitoes.

1897	Anglo-American bacteriologist, THOMAS GILCHRIST, described Gilchrist disease, North American blastomycosis, caused by the soil-borne fungus, *Blastomyces dermatidis*. Once confined to North America, it is now also found in some African countries.
1897	HENRY ROSE CARTER was asked to investigate outbreaks of yellow fever in two isolated hamlets in the upper Mississippi. Here, he made the crucial observation that: 'The fact that yellow fever is not directly transferable through the environment infected by the patient is due to the fact that the material leaving a patient must undergo some change in the environment before it is capable of infecting another man.'
1897	The excision of the apex of the lung as an effective cure for pulmonary tuberculosis was described by THEODORE TUFFIER of France.
1898	HENRI TRIBOULET, a French physician, isolated streptococci from patients with acute rheumatism, and later devised a fecal test for intestinal tuberculosis, which is now obsolete.
1898	NATHAN E. BRILL discovered a previously unrecognized form of the rickettsial disease, typhus, recrudescent or endemic typhus (also called Brill–Zinsser disease, after HANS ZINSSER).
1898	Dutch botanist MARTINUS BEIJERINCK, described 'filterable viruses.'

1898	JAMES CARROLL, an Anglo-American physician, developed a typhoid vaccine which he tried on himself and died from resulting complications nine years later.
1898	A seroagglutination test for the tubercle bacillus was designed by physician, SATURNIN ARLOING.
1898	*Treponema vincentii*, a spirochete found in the throat of patients with Vincent angina, was identified by French bacteriologist, HENRI VINCENT.
1899	DAME ANNIE JEAN MACNAMARA born. An Australian physician who discovered that there was more than one strain of the poliomyelitis virus which paved the way for the development of the Salk vaccine.
1900	HENRY HEAD, an English neurologist, with ALFRED W. CAMPBELL, studied herpes zoster and established that the disease is an inflammation of the posterior nerve ganglia and roots.
1900	Polish bacteriologist J. DANYSZ grew a variant of *Bacillus anthracis*, capable of tolerating five times the normal inhibitory concentration of arsenic.
1900	Smallpox was almost entirely eliminated in England and Prussia.
1900	Belgian physiologist, JULES JEAN BORDET, described complement, a thermolabile component of serum.
1900	Death of American physician, JESSE WILLIAM LAZEAR, who deliberately and fatally allowed a mosquito to bite him during an outbreak of yellow fever in Havana, thus helping to establish the mosquito as a transmitter of the disease.

Dates in Infectious Diseases

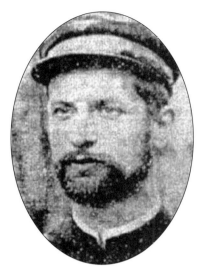

Alexandre Émile
John Yersin
(1863–1943)

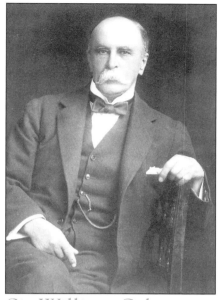

Sir William Osler
(1849–1919)

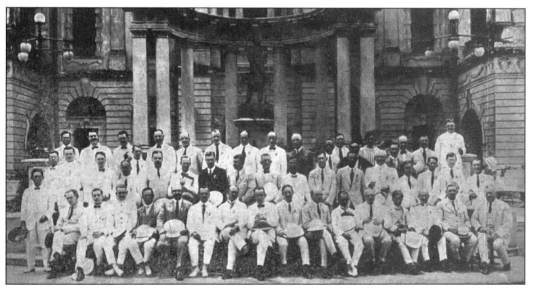

Camille Guérin (1872–1961)
Far Eastern Association of Tropical Medicine Meeting

1900	Between a third and half of all babies born in the USA never saw their 5th birthday. Whooping cough, diphtheria, rheumatic fever and scarlet fever were the major killers.
1900	The Wesbrook classification of diphtheria bacilli was proposed by American physician, FRANK FAIRCHILD WESBROOK of Minneapolis.
1900	The mycelial nature of the fungus in coccidiomycosis was demonstrated by WILLIAM OPHULS and HERBERT C. MOFFIT of America.
1900	CHARLES LOUIS LAVERAN of France described the genus of coccidian protozoa (*Toxoplasma*).
1900	An American team, headed by WATER REED, discovered that yellow fever is transmitted by mosquitoes.
1900	The average life-span was 47 years in the USA.
1901	WILLIAM LEISHMAN identified organisms taken from the spleen of a patient in India who had died from dum-dum fever (later named Leishmaniasis).
1901	The first Nobel Prize for medicine was awarded to EMIL VON BEHRING for his discovery of the first 'reliable weapon' against diphtheria.
1901	Radium in the treatment of tuberculous disease of the skin was first used (with P. BLOCH) by the French dermatologist, HENRI ALEXANDRE DANLOS.

Dates in Infectious Diseases

1902 A swelling of the pneumococcal bacterial capsule when treated with its antiserum (Quellung reaction) was observed by FRED NEUFELD.

1902 The Wellcome Tropical Research Laboratories were formally opened. The center for investigation into tropical diseases was based in Khartoum in the Sudan, and featured a floating laboratory on the River Nile that enabled research and medical teams to reach regions that were not otherwise easily accessible.

1902 American physician, FREDERICK FORCHHEIMER, wrote *Diseases of the Mouth in Children*, and described the Forchheimer sign: a reddish eruption on the soft palate that precedes skin eruption in rubella.

1902 SIR RONALD ROSS of the Indian Medical Service was awarded the Nobel Prize for his work on the life cycle of the malarial parasite and the transmission of malaria. Ross collaborated with PATRICK MANSON who had originally shown that malaria was transmitted by mosquito bites.

1902 CHARLES ROBERT RICHET, a French physiologist, did pioneering work on serum therapy, and coined the term, anaphylaxis, to denote an allergic reaction.

1902 FORD and DUTTON, working in the Gambia, identified *Trypanosoma brucci gambiense*, the parasite in sleeping sickness.

1903 Extensive work on syphilis was carried out by Austrian pathologist, HANS CHIARI.

1903	ALDO CASTELLANI, working in Uganda, found trypanosomes in the cerebrospinal fluid of a patient with sleeping sickness.
1903	SIR ALMROTH EDWARD WRIGHT, an English bacteriologist, developed a typhoid vaccine, worked on parasitic diseases and contributed to the discovery of a thermolabile substance in the serum acting on bacteria during phagocytosis.
1903	DAVID BRUCE identified the tsetse fly as the vector of trypanosomiasis.
1903	Inflammation of the spinal canal (arachnoiditis) was described in a patient as 'meningitis circumscripta spinalis' by WILLIAM GIBSON SPILLER, J.H. MUSSER and EDWARD MARTIN.
1904	FRED NEUFELD, a German bacteriologist, described bacteriotrophins and demonstrated lysis of pneumococci by bile salts.
1904	A spirochete from a genus of tick which causes African relapsing fever (Dutton fever) by transmitting the spirochete, *Borrelia recurrentis*, was identified independently by two groups; ROSS and MILNE in Uganda, and JOSEPH EVERETT DUTTON and JOHN LANCELOT TODD of the Liverpool School of Tropical Medicine in England, in the Congo.
1904	PAUL EHRLICH found an aniline dye that killed South American horsepox bacteria in infected mice.
1904	RAYMOND SABOURAUD, a French dermatologist, developed X-ray treatment for ringworm, attained a

world reputation for his work on ringworm and dermatophytes, and devised the Sabouraud culture medium for pathogenic fungi.

1905 German dermatologist, ERICH HOFFMANN, prepared the serum for the historic discovery of *Treponema pallidum*.

1905 BÉLA SCHICK of Hungary gave the first description of serum disease, and developed the Schick test, a skin test that determines a patient's susceptibility to diphtheria and vulnerability to disease in general (1921).

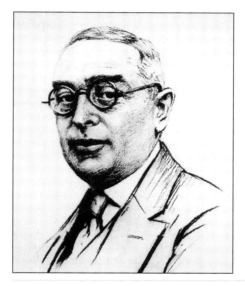

Béla Schick
(1877–1967)

1905 The fungus and causative agent of histoplasmosis (*Histoplasma capsulatum*) was described by American, SAMUEL T. DARLIN.

1905 GEORGE HERBERT HITCHINGS, an American biochemist born. He discovered the folic acid antagonist 2-aminopurine, the anti-malarial pyrimethamine, the anti-leukemia drug 6-mercatopurine, and the immunosuppressant azathioprine.

1905 FRITZ SCHAUDINN, a German protozoologist, discovered the spirochete, *Treponema pallidum*, the causative organism of syphilis, and demonstrated that hookworm infection occurs through the feet.

1905 Scientific evidence for communicability of the polio virus was provided by OTTO IVAR WICKMAN during an epidemic in Sweden.

1905 CLEMENS VON PIRQUET, an Austrian immunologist who coined the term 'allergy', devised the Pirquet test for diagnosis of tuberculosis, where tuberculin was applied through a needle scratch on the skin.

1905 ROBERT KOCH was awarded the Nobel Prize for Physiology or Medicine for his contribution to bacteriology.

1906 Rough and smooth colonies of dysentery bacilli and their particular relevance to antigenic properties, were discovered by JOSEPH ARKWRIGHT, a bacteriologist at the Lister Institute.

1906 AUGUST VON WASSERMANN, German bacteriologist and director of the Institute of Experimental Therapy in Berlin, developed the complementation test for diagnosis of syphilis (Wassermann test).

1906 ALMROTH WRIGHT was knighted in recognition of his work on the protective power of blood against bacteria, the activities of opsonins, and the involvement of the immune system and serum factors. He also developed the first antityphoid inoculation.

Dates in Infectious Diseases

1906   SIMON FLEXNER of the Rockefeller Institute of Medical Research was asked to deal with an outbreak of meningococcal meningitis in New York. He used infected horses as a source of antiserum (Flexner serum) and cut the fatalities to 25%. He also studied 'toxic death' by injecting dog serum into rabbits – an early experiment in anaphylaxis.

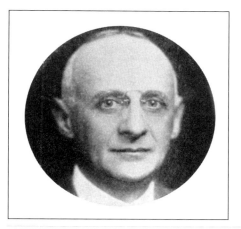

Simon Flexner (1863–1946)

1906   Dengue fever was shown to be transmitted by *Aedes aegypti* (and the Asian tiger mosquito, *A. albopictus*) by THOMAS LANE BANCROFT.

1907   CHARLES LAVERAN of the Pasteur Institute in France was awarded the Nobel Prize for his discovery of the malarial parasite and work on protozoal disease. He also did important work on leishmaniasis, sleeping sickness and kala-azar.

1907   GEORGE FERDINAND WIDAL, a French microbiologist, devised the Widal test for typhoid fever based on the agglutination reaction which showed that the reaction was due to infection rather than immunity.

1907	German microbiologist, STANISLAUS VON PROWAZEK, found cell inclusion bodies in conjunctival cells in trachoma, and postulated that they were collections of virus enveloped by material deposited from the infected cell.
1908	PAUL EHRLICH, a German bacteriologist, and Russian embryologist, ELIE METCHNIKOFF, shared the Nobel Prize for Physiology or Medicine for their contributions to immunity and serum therapy.
1908	KARL LANDSTEINER determined that polio is caused by a virus, not a bacteria.
1908	HOWARD RICKETTS discovered a new class of bacteria, the rickettsiae.
1908	Sulfonamide was synthesized in Austria but its antibacterial properties remained unnoticed until 1930 when it was shown to be an active constituent of Prontosil.
1909	Arachnoiditis, the inflammation of the spinal canal, was described as 'chronic spinal meningitis' by VICTOR HORSLEY.
1909	FRANCIS A. BAINBRIDGE, an English physiologist and bacteriologist, classified various strains of *Salmonella*.
1909	CARLOS CHAGAS of Brazil discovered the protozoan, *Trypanosoma*, and its insect vector causing trypanosomiasis, and the disease was later named after him.
1909	A diagnostic test for meningitis (Brudzinski sign) was described by Polish physician, J. BRUDZINSKI.

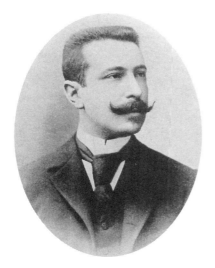

Georges Ferdinand
Isidore Widal
(1862–1929)

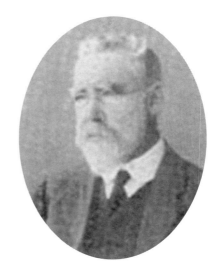

Thomas Lane
Bancroft
(1860–1933)

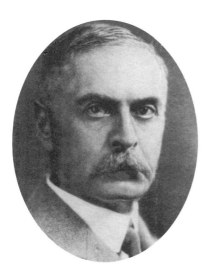

Karl Landsteiner
(1868–1943)

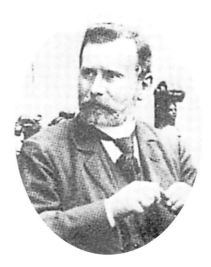

Paul Ehrlich
(1854–1915)

Dates in Infectious Diseases

1909 — ALBERTO BARTON of Peru discovered the bacterium *Bartonella baccilliformis*, found in red blood cells causing Bartonellosis (Peruvian Oroya fever), an acute febrile hemolytic anemia.

1909 — A diagnostic serology test for echinococcus (Weinberg test) was described by Paris physician, MICHEL WEINBERG.

1909 — GEORGE HENRY FALKINER NUTTALL, a pathologist from Johns Hopkins University, introduced trypan as treatment for babesiasis.

1909 — ARVID AFZELIUS of Sweden described a circular skin rash, with a peculiar mode of spreading. He hypothesized that the disease was transmitted by the *Ixodes ricinus* tick.

1910 — A modified Wassermann test for syphilis (Emery test) was devised by English physician, D. WALTER EMERY.

1910 — Salvarsan (neoarsphenamine, or the magic bullet) was developed and used in treatment for syphilis by German bacteriologist and Nobel Prize winner, PAUL EHRLICH, and was later found to be effective in the treatment of relapsing fever and trypanosomiasis. Subsequently, Ehrlich discovered the less toxic neosalvarsan.

1910 — The subcutaneous injection of a controlled amount of tuberculin for the tuberculin test (for diagnosis of tuberculosis) was introduced by French physician, CHARLES MANTOUX.

1910	Boston pathologist, JAMES HOMER WRIGHT, developed Wright stain for megakaryocytes and platelets, and prepared special stains for the malarial parasite.
1910	HUGO SCHOTTMÜLLER, a German professor of medicine, isolated *Streptococcus viridans* from the blood of patients with bacterial endocarditis, having earlier described paratyphoid (1900).
1910	WILLIAM PARKS conclusively proved that the bovine tuberculosis bacillus causes most tuberculosis in children who had ingested unpasteurized milk.
1910	Death of RICKETTS from typhus, the pathologist who first detected the organisms that cause Rocky Mountain spotted fever and louse-borne typhus.
1911	BÉLA SCHICK gave the first description of serum disease and developed the Schick test that determines a patient's vulnerability to disease. He also reduced the death rate from diphtheria by using his test in which a small amount of diphtheria toxin is injected into the skin.
1911	FRANCIS PEYTON ROUS discovered the Rous sarcoma virus (RSV) in chickens, the first cancer shown to be caused by a virus. The human immunodeficiency virus (HIV) is a member of the same retrovirus family.
1911	CHARLES HENRI NICOLLE, a French physician and director of the Pasteur Institute in Tunis, identified the body louse as a transmitter of typhus fever for which he was awarded the Nobel Prize for Physiology or Medicine (1928).

1912	Azotemia produced by an extrarenal cause such as cholera (prerenal uremia) was observed by GEORGE FROIN and PIERRE MARIE of Paris, France.
1912	Melioidosis, a glanders-like disease, was described by surgeons ALFRED WHITMORE and C.S. KRISHNASWAMI, who carried out their studies in India.
1912	British physician, SIR LEONARD ROGERS, first gave emetine injections for amebic dysentery and hepatitis, advocated intravenous saline in the treatment of dehydration due to cholera, and wrote *Fevers in the Tropics*.
1913	AUGUSTE ROLLIER, a Swiss physician, advocated the use of increasing doses of sunlight in the treatment of tuberculosis.
1913	The Lange test for cerebrospinal fluid using gold chloride to detect various forms of cerebrospinal syphilis, was devised by CARL FRIEDRICH LANGE of Berlin.
1913	MAURICE FAVRE, a French dermatologist, described lymphogranuloma venereum (Favre disease), which he separated from other venereal diseases.
1913	CHARLES ROBERT RICHET, a French physiologist, who did pioneering work on serum therapy, was awarded the Nobel Prize.
1914	Mumps, a disease known since ancient times, was only established with British bacteriologist MERVYN HENRY GORDON'S discovery that it was caused by a filterable agent.

1914	WILHELM GENNERICH, a German dermatologist, introduced treatment of neurosyphilis by intraspinal injections of arsephenamine and designed a special device for forcing the salvarsanized cerebrospinal fluid into the brain.
1914	*Infection and Resistance* was written by New York bacteriologist and immunologist, HANS ZINSSER, who worked on allergy, virus size, typhus and causes of rheumatic fevers.
1914	Experimental proof that rubella (German measles) is caused by a virus was provided by ALFRED FABIAN HESS of America.
1914	The viral etiology of the illness 'common cold' was demonstrated by German bacteriologist, WALTHER KRUSE.
1915	The causative agent of Weil disease, *Leptospira icterohemorrhagia*, was identified independently by RYUKICHI INADO and YUTAKA IDO of Japan.
1915	THOMAS HUCKLE WELLER born. A virologist from Michigan who worked on *Schistosoma* and poliomyelitis cell cultivation, and shared the Nobel Prize for his work on the chickenpox and shingles virus.
1916	FREDERICK CHAPMAN ROBBINS born. An Alabama physiologist and pediatrician who succeeded in cultivating the poliomyelitis virus, an important step in the development of the polio vaccine.
1916	An agglutinin reaction for diagnosis of typhus (Weil–Felix reaction) was devised by Polish

bacteriologist, ARTHUR FELIX and German physician, EDMUND WEIL. The test was later applied to differentiate between various rickettsial diseases.

1917   The epidemic 'encephalitis lethargica' (von Economo disease) was described by French surgeon, JEAN CRUCHET and Austrian neurologist CONSTANTIN VON ECONOMO. In 1918 Economo showed that a submicroscopic virus was the cause of infection.

1917   The Spanish flu, the most lethal influenza pandemic, killed over 20 million people. First World War troop movements aided its spread.

1917   MICHAEL HEIDELBERGER and JACOBS reported that sulfanilic acid killed bacteria. It was some time before the compound was used because bacteria were not considered susceptible to chemotherapy.

1917   JULIUS WAGNER-JUAREGG infected patients with malaria and showed that it could cure many symptoms of syphilis.

1917   A vaccine was developed against Rocky Mountain spotted fever.

1917   Facial paralysis, painful ears, vesicular eruption of the oropharynx, due to herpes zoster and infection of the geniculate ganglion (Ramsay Hunt syndrome), was described by American neurologist, JAMES RAMSAY HUNT.

1918   GERTRUDE BELLE ELION born. An American biochemist who worked on the synthesis of compounds that

Dates in Infectious Diseases

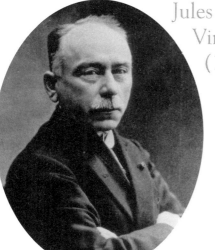

Jules Jean Baptiste Vincent Bordet (1870–1961)

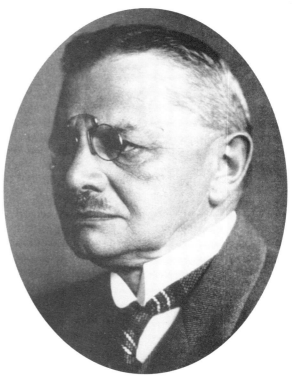

Alfons Maria Jakob (1884–1931)

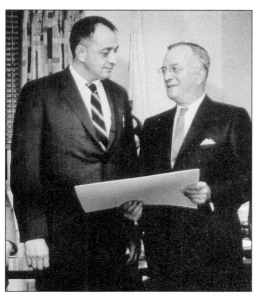

Robert Good (b. 1922)

	inhibited DNA synthesis. She produced the antiviral compound acyclovir and compounds that had potential in cancer therapy.
1918	SIR ANDREW BALFOUR of Edinburgh made important contributions to the study of tropical diseases, founded the Museum of Tropical Diseases and was the first director of Wellcome Research Laboratories.
1918	In the First World War epidemic typhus on the Eastern Front killed at least three million soldiers.
1919	JULES BORDET received the Nobel Prize for his work on immunity factors in blood serum. Together with his brother-in-law, OCTAVE GENGOU, he also discovered the whooping cough bacillus and prepared a vaccine against it, and isolated the bacteria for bovine peripneumonia and for avian diphtheria.
1919	WILHELM HIS JUNIOR, a German physician, described trench fever (calling it Volhynia fever).
1920	Chaulmoogra oil, obtained from the seed of the kalaw tree, was introduced to the west by FREDERICK JOHN MOURAT as a treatment for leprosy. Indian Hindus had recognized its properties thousands of years before.
1920	A syndrome of dementia accompanied by pyramidal and extrapyramidal signs which usually occur after middle age (Creutzfeldt–Jakob disease) was described by HANS CREUTZFELDT and ALFONS JAKOB.
1920	CARL FRIEDRICH MEYER of the University of California introduced the name *Brucella* for bacteria which caused Malta fever, in honor of its discoverer SIR DAVID BRUCE.

1921   CAMILLE GUÉRIN and L.C. ALBERT CALMETTE began experiments to produce acquired immunity by injecting attenuated tuberculous bacilli, leading to the Bacille Calmette–Guérin vaccination (BCG).

1921   WILHELM ROEHL studied the properties of an azo dye derivative and developed Germanin for treatment of sleeping sickness.

1921   ERNEST GOODPASTURE and TALBERT suggested that cytomegalia could be due to a viral agent.

1922   The Kahn test, a diagnostic precipitin test for diagnosis of syphilis, was devised by REUBEN LEON KHAN, a bacteriologist at the University of Michigan School of Medicine.

1922   ROBERT GOOD born. He was director of the Sloan-Kettering Institute for Cancer Research in New York and showed the importance of the Bursa of Fabricius and the B and T lymphocytes. He pioneered bone-marrow transplantation and is immortalized in the Good Syndrome, a gammaglobulinemia associated with thymoma and deficiencies in both humoral and cellular immunity which results in repeated fungal, viral, and pyogenic infections.

1923   The fungus causing thrush, *Candida albicans*, was named by CHRISTINE BERKHOUT of the University of Delft.

1923   Hemolytic streptococci was shown as the cause of scarlet fever by GEORGE FREDERICK DICK and his wife GLADYS ROWENA DICK of the Johns Hopkins School of Medicine, and subsequently a skin test (Dick test) was devised a year later.

1923	ADRIAN STOKES, an American pathologist, found the specific virus of yellow fever, and died from it during his experimentation.
1923	First vaccinations for diphtheria.
1923	Vaccination against tuberculosis, the BCG vaccine, is developed.
1924	ARVID JOHAN WALLGREN from Sweden described aseptic meningitis, acute lymphocytic choriomeningitis.
1924	Somatic antigens were first identified in cases of *Salmonella typhi* infection by Polish bacteriologist ARTHUR FELIX.
1924	Tryparsamide is introduced for treatment of sleeping sickness.
1925	The infectiousness of herpes zoster was first demonstrated by German physician, KARL KUNDRATITZ.
1925	Photomicrography was first applied to the study of bacteria and viruses by JOSEPH EDWIN BARNARD.
1925	British bacteriologist, MERVYN HENRY GORDON, described a precipitin test for differentiating between smallpox and chickenpox, and published an important study of the viruses of vaccinia and variola.
1925	Bistovol (bismuth stovarsol) was prepared by C. LEVADETTI for the treatment of syphilis.

Dates in Infectious Diseases

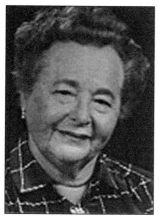

Gertrude Belle Elion
Nobel Laureate Physiology
or Medicine 1988

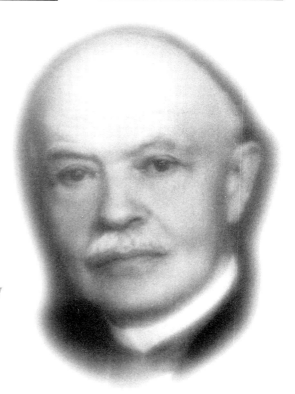

Charles Jules Henri Nicolle
(1866–1936)

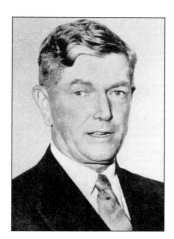

Sir Frank
Macfarlane Burnet
(1899–1985)

Sir Alexander Fleming
(1881–1955)

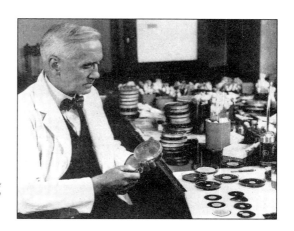

1926 Reports on the treatment of erysipelas with antistreptococcal serum were given by American bacteriologist, KONRAD E. BIRKHANG.

1926 THEOBALD SMITH of New York elucidated the tick as vector of Texas Cattle Fever, distinguished human from bovine tuberculosis, developed bacteriological techniques for examining milk, water and sewage, and improved vaccines for several diseases. He also formulated the principle of the antibody–antigen reaction.

1926 First vaccinations for pertussis.

1927 GASTON RAMON used formaldehyde-inactivated diphtheria toxin or tetanus toxin to stimulate production of active immunity. A combination of these two inactivated toxins is now used routinely to immunize children against diphtheria and tetanus.

1927 Scottish bacteriologist, SIR ALEXANDER FLEMING, discovered that penicillium mold inhibited the growth of staphylococci. A 93% decline in mortality due to pneumonia in children was reported in 2000, largely due to penicillin.

1927 Austrian neurologist, JULIUS WAGNER-JAUREGG, received the Nobel Prize for his work on fever therapy for late stage syphilis and other diseases.

1927 PHILIP DRINKER and LOUIS SHAW develop the iron lung, widely used for polio victims.

1927 WADE HAMPTON FROST developed statistical methods, including cohort analysis of mortality data and use of morbidity surveys, and development of life tables that took epidemiology from a 'descriptive' to an 'analytical' discipline. He developed the well known Reed–Frost model of susceptibility and probability of individual infection through contact. He used these methods to study poliomyelitis (1913), common cold (1932) and tuberculosis (1933).

1927 First vaccinations for tetanus.

1928 A local skin reaction to the filtrate of typhus bacillus culture (Schwartzmann phenomenon) was described by New York physician GREGORY SCHWARTZMANN.

1928 CHARLES HENRI NICOLLE, a French physician and director of the Pasteur Institute in Tunis, was awarded the Nobel Prize for his work on transmission of typhus by body lice.

1928 British physician FREDERICK GRIFFITH found that extracts of a pathogenic strain of pneumococcus could transform a harmless strain into a pathogenic one.

1930 The Lübeck disaster took the lives of a large number of children in Germany, when the BCG vaccination for tuberculosis was contaminated.

1930 KARL LANDSTEINER was awarded the Nobel Prize for his work on distinguishing human blood into three groups: A, B and C (later called O). He also demonstrated transmission of poliomyelitis by intraspinal injection and later isolated the virus. He devised techniques to couple simple compounds to proteins and showed antibody specificity to an antigen.

1930	An epidemic febrile infectious disease on the Danish island of Bornholm was described by EJNER OLUF SORENSON as Bornholm disease.
1930	Swedish chemist, ARNE WILHELM TISELIUS, isolated several viruses and separated and identified amino acids, sugars and other molecules using activated charcoal, silica, cellulose and ion exchange chromatography.
1931	Post-streptococcal arthritis following tonsillitis was noted as being due to an allergy to bacterial products rather than bacterial toxins by FREDERICK JOHN POYNTON.
1931	WILLIAM ELFORD proved that virus could be trapped in an ultrafilter.
1931	Australian immunologist, SIR FRANK MACFARLANE BURNET, perfected a technique of growing virus in eggs.
1931	WILLIAM WELLS, of the Harvard School of Public Health, developed an instrument for bacterial examination of air. He also investigated droplet nuclei of infection and the use of UV radiation in destroying such sources of infection.
1931	The virus from the human skin in herpes lesions was grown on the chorioallantois membrane of chicks by ERNEST GOODPASTURE and ANDERSON. This provided a means of virus culture for vaccine production.
1931	HAMILTON SMITH born. An American molecular biologist who discovered endonucleases in bacteria that can split the DNA of invading phage particles and inactivate them.

Dates in Infectious Diseases

1932 Löffler syndrome (pulmonary symptoms and eosinophilic infiltration of the lung secondary to helminthic infection) was described by WILHELM LÖFFLER of Switzerland.

1932 Introduction of the antimalarial drug, atebrin.

1932 The presence of heterophilic antibodies in infectious mononucleosis (glandular fever) was shown by Americans, JOHN RODMAN PAUL and WALLS WILLARD BUNNEL.

1933 A classification of pathogenic hemolytic streptococci based on serology and pathogenicity (Lancefield group) was proposed by a bacteriologist from the Rockefeller Institute in New York, REBECCA CRAIGHILL LANCEFIELD. The previously named *Diplococcus rheumaticus*, the causative bacteria of rheumatic fever, was identified as Streptococcus group A in 1940.

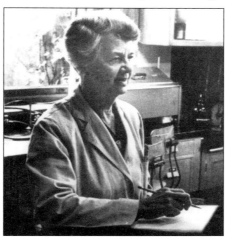

Rebecca Craighill Lancefield (1895–1981)

1933 A fibrinolytic substance from group A beta-hemolytic streptococcus was isolated by Baltimore physicians, WILLIAM SMITH TILLET and R.L. GARNER.

Dates in Infectious Diseases

1933 The causative virus of St Louis encephalitis (mosquito-carried arbovirus, named after an epidemic in St Louis, USA) and lymphocytic choriomeningitis was identified by CHARLES ARMSTRONG.

1934 *Rats, Lice and History* was published by HANS ZINSSER. He noted that wars 'are only the terminal operations engaged in by those remnants of the armies which have survived the camp epidemics.'

1934 Polish-American microbiologist, ALBERT BRUCE SABIN, researched vaccines against Japanese B encephalitis and dengue fever (1945).

1935 WENDELL STANLEY showed that viruses could be crystallized without losing their ability to produce disease.

1935 First vaccinations for yellow fever, developed by MAX THEILER.

1935 German biochemist, GERHARD DOMAGK, discovered the antibiotic and red azo dye, Protonsil. This contains sulfanilamide, the first antibacterial substance to give protection against streptococcal infection. He also introduced thiosemicarbazone for tuberculosis.

1935 The National Foundation for Infantile Paralysis, the first center in the world for research into polio, was established in America.

1936 SIR PHILLIPE BEDSON, a London bacteriologist, devised a laboratory diagnosis for lymphogranuloma venereum, through skin testing with an antigen.

1936	J.J. BITTNER demonstrated that cancer can be transmitted in mice through milk, thus suggesting that some viruses can cause cancer.
1937	Q fever, originally named 'Q' to denote query as the causative agent (*Coxiella burnetii*) was unknown, was observed by EDWARD HOLBROOK DERRICK in Australia, after an outbreak of febrile illness amongst meat and cattle workers in Brisbane.
1937	A disorder characterized by thrombocytopenic purpura and susceptibility to staphylococcal infection due to antibody deficiency (Wiskott-Aldrich syndrome), was described by German pediatrician, ALFRED WISKOTT.
1937	Orogenital ulceration (Behçet syndrome) was described by Turkish dermatologist, HALUSHI BEHÇET, who carried out long and extensive studies on this disease, and wrote the book *Syphilis and Related Skin Diseases*.
1937	Early descriptions of ardent fever were found consistent with blackwater fever by JOHN WILLIAM STEPHENS.
1937	EDWIN SCHULTZ used a polio vaccine nasal spray on 5,000 children in Toronto. Several children lost their sense of smell permanently.
1937	The antibacterial sulfa drug, sulfapyridine was developed.
1938	The Laidlaw-Green hypothesis that postulates that viruses arose from larger microorganisms due to their redundant parasitic mode of life, was proposed

independently by SIR PATRICK PLAYFAIR LAIDLAW of Cambridge and R.P. GREEN.

1938 GLADWIN ALBERT HURST BUTTLE and co-workers introduced dapsone as a treatment for leprosy.

1938 Coxsackie virus was named after Coxsackie in New York where it was identified. Coxsackie virus B4 (a relative of the poliovirus) was isolated from the pancreas of a child who died accidentally shortly after the onset of diabetes.

1939 An effective vaccine against whooping cough was introduced by PEARL KENDRICK and GRACE ELDERLING.

1939 MAX THEILER, a South African-born American bacteriologist who worked on amebic dysentery and yellow fever, produced vaccine from attenuated live yellow fever virus that led to the development of the 17D vaccine for yellow fever.

1939 RENÉ DUBOS, a French bacteriologist working in America, isolated one of the first antibacterial substances from *Bacillus brevis* and named it tyrothricin.

1939 CHARLES RAMMELKAMP joined the Commission on Acute Respiratory Diseases. He studied the epidemiology of streptococcal infections and the clinical application and mode of action of antimicrobial agents.

1939 GERALD DOMAGK was awarded the Nobel Prize for his discovery of Prontosil.

Dates in Infectious Diseases

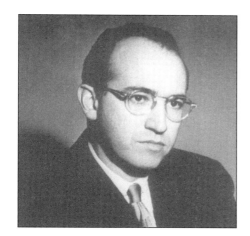

Albert Bruce Sabin
(1906–1993)

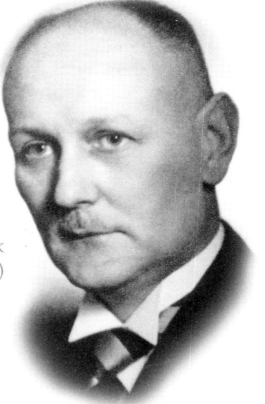

Gerhard Domagk
(1895–1964)

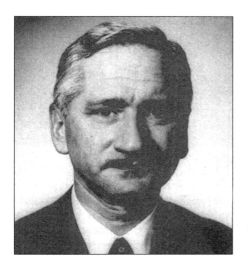

Jonas Edward Salk
(b 1914)

Dates in Infectious Diseases

1939 The development of penicillin as an antibiotic, mainly due to the work of HOWARD WALTER FLOREY and ERNST CHAIN at the Sir William Dunn School of Pathology at Oxford, England.

1939 DDT was synthesized by PAUL MÜLLER in Switzerland.

1940 ROBIN WEISS born. An English molecular biologist and head of the Imperial Cancer Research Chester Beatty Laboratory, who works on the role of retroviruses in causing cancer and on the HIV virus and its mechanism of entry into the cell.

1940 The influenza B virus was isolated independently by THOMAS FRANCIS and THOMAS PLEINES MAGILL.

1940 New York bacteriologist, REBECCA CRAIGHILL LANCEFIELD, classified strains of streptococci that have rheumatogenic capability in rheumatic fever.

1940 HOWARD FLOREY and ERNST CHAIN showed that penicillin protected mice against a number of bacteria.

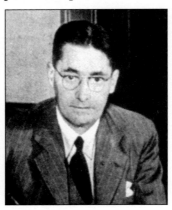

Howard Walter Florey
(1895–1968)

1940	American bacteriologist, HAROLD RAE COX, prepared a typhus vaccine (Cox vaccine) from yolk-sac culture of rickettsial species.
1940	SISTER ELIZABETH KENNY developed rehabilitation techniques for polio victims, using hot packs and re-education of muscles.
1940	SELMAN WAKSMAN and his team isolated an effective anti-TB antibiotic, actinomycin. In the following year he coined the term 'antibiotic.'
1941	The Hirst test, used to detect viruses or their corresponding antibodies, was devised by New York physician, GEORGE KEBLE HIRST.
1941	A link was established between rubella and birth deformities.
1943	A pure form of cardiolipin was obtained from beef heart by MARY CANDACE PANGBORN, and was introduced as an agent for serological diagnosis of syphilis.
1943	Penicillin was first used in the treatment of syphilis by JOHN FRIEND MAHONEY and colleagues, of the US Public Health Service.
1943	The antibiotic bacitracin was isolated from *Bacillus subtilis* from a compound fracture in a girl named MARGARET TRACY.
1943	Successful trial of killed-virus polio vaccine developed by JONAS SALK and THOMAS FRANCIS.

1943	Hepatitis B (HBV), the virus responsible for serum hepatitis, was first shown to be present in some batches of human pooled serum by FREDERICK OGDEN MACCALLUM and DENNIS JOHN BAUER.
1943	In the Second World War, typhus was very active on the Eastern Front but an outbreak in Naples and post-war outbreaks in Germany were cut short by the new insecticide, DDT.
1944	An outbreak of pneumonia, due to histoplasma infection from a storm cellar, occurred in Oklahoma.
1944	T. DUCKETT JONES of Massachusetts General Hospital, published his classic paper, 'The Diagnosis of Rheumatic Fever', describing the major and minor manifestations that could be used for accurate diagnosis. The criteria subsequently became associated with his name and revolutionized diagnosis.
1944	THEODORE OSWALD AVERY of New York, a pioneer in molecular biology and immunochemistry, discovered the type III antigen of pneumococcus and demonstrated its antigenic functions. He wrote 'Induction of Transformation by a Deoxyribonucleic Acid Fraction Isolated from Pneumococcus Type lll.'
1944	ALBERT SABIN isolated the virus that causes dengue fever and showed that it belongs to the *Flaviviridae* virus family. There are four known serotypes of dengue virus: DEN-1, DEN-2, DEN-3, and DEN-4.
1944	SELMAN WAKSMAN isolated streptomycin from *Streptomyces griseus*, and showed that it combined maximal inhibition of *M. tuberculosis* with relatively

low toxicity. On November 20 the antibiotic was administered to a critically ill TB patient. The disease was arrested, the bacteria disappeared from his sputum, and he made a rapid recovery.

1945 A.M.M. PAYNE reported mild cases of hepatitis in patients with amebic dysentery, known as amebic hepatitis.

1945 COLIN MACLEOD, OSWALD AVERY and MACLYN MCCARTY, of the Rockefeller Institute, published their work on pneumococcus They elucidated the role of deoxyribonucleic acid as the genetic determinant of the pneumococcal capsular carbohydrate. Macleod also studied pneumococcal pneumonia and produced the type-specific antiserum and introduced treatment with sulfonamides. Together with HEIDELBERGER, HODGES and BERNHARD, he provided the first clear demonstration of the prophylactic value of vaccines made from purified pneumococcal capsular carbohydrates.

1945 F.S.H. CURD and co-workers synthesized paludrine, or proguanil, and tested it against avian malaria.

1945 SIR HOWARD FLOREY, ERNST CHAIN and ALEXANDER FLEMING shared the Nobel Prize for Physiology or Medicine for their work on antibiotics.

1945 RENÉ DUBOS published his famous monograph, *The Bacterial Cell*.

1945 HIMSHAW and FELDMAN proved the effectiveness of streptomycin in the treatment of tuberculosis. This was one of the earliest controlled trials.

1946	American bacteriologist, JOHN FRANKLIN ENDERS, cultivated the polio virus in human tissue at his laboratory for poliomyelitis, which led to the development of the polio vaccine.
1946	JOSHUA LEDERBERG'S studies on sexual conjugation in *Escherichia coli* led to the construction of chromosome maps.
1946	German biophysicist and pioneer in genetics of the phage, MAX DELBRUCK, discovered that viruses can exchange genetic material to create new types of viruses.
1946	Nitrofuranotoin, an oral urinary antibacterial compound developed from nitrofuran drugs, was introduced by M. DODD.
1946	Cardiolipin antigen was used in the serological test for diagnosis of syphilis.
1947	A cholera epidemic in Egypt killed 20,500 of 30,000 people infected.
1947	Glaxo developed the first combined whooping cough and diphtheria vaccine, and Crystapen, a stable crystalline form of penicillin.
1948	Swedish chemist, ARNE WILHELM TISELIUS was awarded the Nobel Prize for Chemistry for his work on protein analysis and development of ion exchange chromatography.
1948	The Coxsackie virus was isolated from the feces of two children during their acute phase of poliomyelitis in

Coxsackie, New York, by American pathologist, GILBERT DALLDORF and GRACE MARY SICKLES.

1948   Glaxo developed streptomycin for TB treatment, and Wellcome developed polymixin anti-bacterials.

1948   The World Health Organization was formed.

1948   The National Institutes of Health were established in the USA.

1948   The National Health Service was inaugurated in Britain.

1948   Cephalosporins were isolated from *Cephalosporium acremonium* by BROTZU. Discovery of the nucleus of cephalosporin in the 1960s permitted Glaxo to produce semisynthetic derivatives which are active against a wide range of bacteria.

1949   The molecular structure of penicillin was first elucidated by DOROTHY CROWFOOT HODGKIN, an English biochemist who received the Nobel Prize for Chemistry (1964) in recognition of her achievements.

1949   The causative fungus of histoplasmosis was isolated from soil by American mycologist, CHESTER EMMONS.

1949   Australian neurologist, SIR HUGH WILLIAM BELL CAIRNS, introduced intrathecal administration of penicillin in the treatment of pneumococcal meningitis. He gave the first description of hydrocephalus after obstruction of the flow of cerebrospinal fluid secondary to tuberculous meningitis.

1949	BENJAMIN DUGGAR discovered the first tetracycline antibiotic, aureomycin.
1949	The Treponema immobilization test for the diagnosis of syphilis was devised by ROBERT ARMSTRONG NELSON and MANFRED MARTIN MAYER.
1949	PETER MEDAWAR discovered the ability of the immune system to accept foreign cells.
1950	The first few cases of severe lymphopenia with extensive candida infection in infancy (combined immunodeficiency) were described in Switzerland.
1950	Life expectancy reached 68 years and this decline in mortality was mainly ascribable to improvements in treatment of infectious diseases.
1950	ROBERT DEBRÉ of France described 'cat scratch fever', characterized by fever and lymphadenopathy.
1951	American geneticist, NORTON DAVID ZINDER, studied mutants of *Salmonella* and described bacterial transduction via a phage.
1951	MAX THEILER was awarded the Nobel Prize for development of the first attenuated virus vaccine for yellow fever.
1952	Daraprim (pyrimethamine) anti-malarial was developed by Wellcome.
1952	DOROTHY HORSTMANN showed that the polio virus entered the bloodstream and that antibodies were also present, thus presenting the possibility of vaccination.

Dates in Infectious Diseases

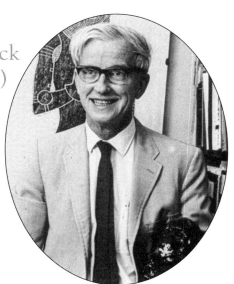

Max Delbruck
(1906–1981)

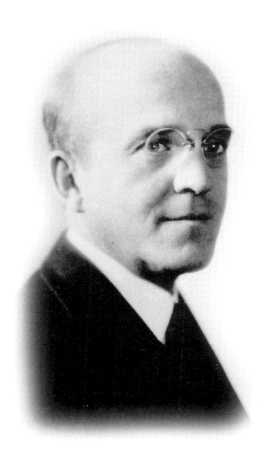

Theodore Oswald Avery
(1877–1955)

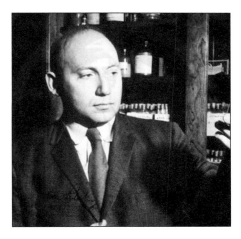

Joshua Lederberg
(b 1925)

Dates in Infectious Diseases

1952 The anti-tuberculous properties of iso-nicotinic acid hydrazide were independently announced by FOX in the USA and a group of German scientists.

1952 Nearly 200,000 Americans contracted polio, and 20,000 died. JONAS SALK tested the killed-virus vaccine at Watson home in Leetsdale, PA. The virus had to be cultured in live monkeys.

1952 The macrolide antibiotic, erythromycin, was discovered by McGUIRE and colleagues in *Streptomyces erythreus*.

1952 SELMAN ABRAHAM WAKSMAN, American microbiologist, received the Nobel Prize for his work in the treatment of tuberculosis with streptomycin.

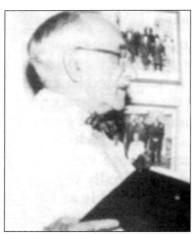

Selman Abraham Waksman (1888–1973)

1953 Only 100 people were affected by polio in the USA following the introduction of the Salk vaccine. SABIN persuaded the Soviets to use his vaccine, which saved a similar number of lives.

1953	Adenovirus was discovered by WALLACE PRESCOTT ROWE, and after further research, more antigenic types and strains were found.
1953	Glaxo produced a tablet form of penicillin, and a triple-antigen vaccine for diphtheria, whooping cough and tetanus.
1953	Discovery of Gentian Violet (Crystal Violet) as chemoprophylactic agent against *Trypanosoma cruzi*-infected blood for transfusion.
1954	The Nobel Prize was awarded to JOHN FRANKLIN ENDERS, THOMAS WELLER and FREDERICK ROBBINS of Boston for their culture of the polio virus.
1954	American physician and founder of the Institute of Medicine of the National Academy of Science, WALSH MCDERMOTT, introduced pyrazinamide in combination with isoniazid as first-line treatment for tuberculosis.
1955	The broad-spectrum antibiotic cycloserine isolated from *Streptomyces orchidaceus*.
1955	Injectable Polio Vaccine (IPV) introduced. Salk's killed-virus polio vaccine was declared 90% effective and safe.
1956	Cardiac involvement by Coxsackie B virus was recognized in newborn infants in Johannesburg by S.N. JAVETT and colleagues.
1956	Vancomycin was developed from the soil fungus, *Streptomyces orientalis*. This inhibits growth of many sensitive Gram-positive bacteria that are resistant to penicillins.

1957	DANIEL BOVET, head of the Laboratory of Therapeutic Chemistry at the Pasteur Institute in Paris; was awarded the Nobel Prize for his work on the treatment of allergies and development of sulfa drugs, and the way in which substances affect and interact with an invading organism.
1957	Pandemic of so-called Asian flu. This started in southwest China, then spread through the Pacific. Mortality was about 0.25%.
1957	ABERT SABIN'S weakened live virus polio vaccine was introduced.
1957	American virologist, DANIEL CARLETON GAJDUSEK, identified a form of spongiform encephalopathy (kuru) amongst the cannibal Fore tribe of Papua New Guinea.
1958	The first success of griseofulvin against fungal infection in humans was recorded by JAMES CLARK GENTLES at Kings College Hospital, London.
1958	At the instigation of the Soviet Union before the World Health Assembly, attempts were started to eradicate smallpox. At that time, the disease claimed two million lives each year.
1958	American biochemist, ARTHUR BECK PARDEE, and JACQUES LUCIEN MONOD started work on the lac operon of *Escherichia coli*.
1958	The virus of Argentine hemorrhagic fever was isolated and found to be immunologically related to a virus called Tacaribe which had been recovered from bats in Trinidad.

Dates in Infectious Diseases

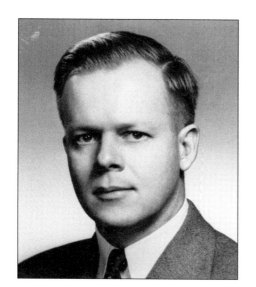

Thomas
Huckle Weller
(b 1915)

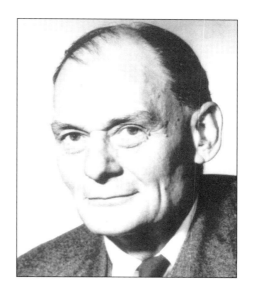

John
Franklin Enders
(1897–1985)

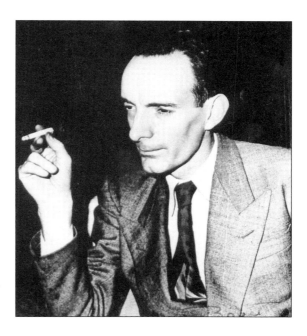

Daniel Bovet
(1907–1992)

1959	Cardiac and renal involvement with pneumonia due to a virus (Lassa fever) was named after Lassa in Nigeria where the disease was first described.
1959	BATCHELOR and colleagues, at the Beecham laboratories, isolated the penicillin nucleus, 6-APA, the precursor for semisynthetic penicillin derivatives, such as methicillin and ampicillin. They synthesized penicillin in the laboratory.
1960	The clonal theory of antibody production, developed by SIR FRANK MACFARLANE BURNET of Australia, earned him the Nobel Prize (shared with PETER MEDAWAR). He also identified the causative rickettsial organism in Q fever, *Coxiella burnetti*.
1960	THOMAS WELLER and co-workers proposed the term cytomegalovirus and subsequently isolated CMV from the urine of infants with generalized disease. CMV has become a common opportunistic pathogen in immunocompromised patients.
1960	*Staphylococcus aureus* was shown to be a major cause of hospital infections.
1961	Pandemic of cholera starts in Indonesia. This pandemic was the seventh recorded.
1961	The American Medical Association endorsed the use of the SABIN oral polio vaccine.
1962	The measles vaccine was developed by American bacteriologist and Nobel Prize winner, JOHN FRANKLIN ENDERS of Connecticut.

Dates in Infectious Diseases

1962 Oral Polio Vaccine (OPV) introduced.

1964 A previously unknown lipoprotein, Australia antigen, was detected by New York biochemist BARUCH SAMUEL BLUMBERG.

1964 The causative organism of infectious mononucleosis (Epstein-Barr virus) was discovered by London microbiologist, SIR MICHAEL ANTHONY EPSTEIN and YVONNE M. BARR. This was the first virus to be associated with cancer.

1964 DOROTHY CROWFOOT HODGKIN, an English biochemist, received the Nobel Prize for Chemistry in recognition of her achievements in elucidating the molecular structure of penicillin.

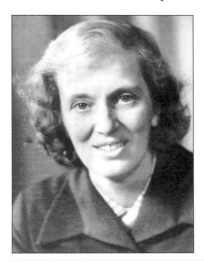

Dorothy Crowfoot Hodgkin
(1910–1994)

1965 Lupoid hepatitis, better known as active chronic hepatitis and accompanied by markers of autoimmune disease, was described by I.R. MACKAY, S. WEIDEN and J. HASKER.

1965	ROBERT BURNS WOODWARD of Boston received the Nobel Prize for Chemistry for his work in synthesizing the antimalarial drug, quinine, cortisone, cholesterol, lysergic acid, reserpine, and chlorophyll.
1965	Measles vaccine was introduced.
1966	Mitochondrial antibodies were demonstrated in 98% of patients with primary biliary cirrhosis, 31% with cryptogenic cirrhosis and 28% with active chronic hepatitis, by DEBORAH DONIACH.
1966	Kuru was experimentally transferred to chimpanzees.
1967	Marburg disease, an acute febrile illness with high mortality similar to that caused by Ebola virus, was reported from Marburg in Germany.
1967	The program for smallpox eradication began, under the direction of the American, DONALD HENDERSON working for the United Nations.
1967	First vaccinations for mumps.
1967	Large-scale measles vaccination program undertaken in Gambia when FOEGE and colleagues administered vaccine in a country-wide campaign. By 1972, indigenous measles was entirely absent from the Gambia. However, due to inability to sustain immunization coverage, the situation has reverted to pre-campaign levels.
1968	Pandemics of so-called Hong Kong flu. The epidemics of 1957 and 1968 are estimated to have killed 1.5 million people. Vaccination is now practiced in several

countries for people deemed to be at risk. However, the surface of the influenza virus is unstable and frequently mutates, which makes any immunity temporary.

1968 J. SHULMAN showed that mice could be infected by airborne transmission of the influenza virus.

1968 Septrin (co-trimoxazole) anti-bacterial introduced by Wellcome. GEORGE HITCHINGS and GERTRUDE ELION synthesized trimethoprim, which was later combined with a sulfamide to form a broad-spectrum systemic antibacterial agent that became a leading anti-bacterial treatment worldwide.

1969 A vaccine for hepatitis was introduced by American biochemist, BARUCH SAMUEL BLUMBERG.

1969 Isolation of Lassa virus from the blood of a missionary nurse in Jos, Nigeria. The virions of Lassa virus were found to be the same as those of LCM, Machupo, Junin and other arenaviruses.

1969 Glaxo launched Ceporex, their first oral cephalosporin antibiotic.

1970 The viral DNA polymerase enzyme which translates into RNA (reverse transcriptase) was discovered independently by American molecular biologist, DAVID BALTIMORE, and virologist, HOWARD MARTIN TEMIN.

1970 First vaccinations for rubella.

1970 EDWARD H. KASS published 'Infectious Diseases and Social Change' in which he discussed seven major infectious diseases in relation not only to modern medical treatment but also to the prevailing socioeconomic conditions, arguing that the latter were paramount in determining deaths.

1970 Plasmids were discovered and shown to be the method by which bacteria evade antibiotics in unpredictable ways.

1971 Wellcome launched a rubella vaccine.

1972 RODNEY PORTER and GERALD EDELMAN shared the Nobel Prize for their discoveries concerning 'the chemical structure of antibodies'. Porter and Edelman showed that the antibody molecule is composed of two pairs of chains, two so-called 'light' and 'heavy' chains, linked by a number of sulfur bridges.

1972 Scientists at Beecham discovered amoxicillin and launched Amoxil, particularly useful in treating bacterial infections such as ear and throat infections in young children. Amoxycillin became the world's most widely used antibiotic.

1973 STANLEY COHEN, ANNIE CHANG, ROBERT HELLING and HERBERT BOYER demonstrated recombinant DNA technology.

1973 Discovery of the Rotavirus, a major cause of infantile diarrhea.

1974 The World Health Organization Immunology of Leprosy program started. Using leprosy bacilli grown in armadillos, they developed a purified vaccine that protects mice against infection. Leprosy affects 12 to 13 million people, mostly in developing countries.

Dates in Infectious Diseases

1974 Possible transmission of Creutzfeldt–Jakob disease to humans was noted.

1974 Smallpox eliminated from India.

1974 The Expanded Program on Immunization of the WHO was created. Six diseases were chosen: tuberculosis, diphtheria, neonatal tetanus, whooping cough, poliomyelitis and measles. Selection was made on the basis of a high burden of disease and the availability of well-tried vaccines at an affordable price. A further three vaccines were added later: yellow fever, hepatitis B, and measles, mumps and rubella combined vaccine (MMR).

1975 Lyme disease was first characterized in patients from Lyme in Connecticut, where a cluster of cases was discovered.

1975 Monoclonal antibodies were produced by an Argentinean-born immunologist, CESAR MILSTEIN, and GEORGE KOHLER at the Medical Research Council Laboratory of Molecular Biology in England. They produced hybridomas that produce specific antibodies that survive indefinitely in tissue culture.

1975 Discovery of Parvovirus B19, the cause of aplastic crisis in chronic hemolytic anemia.

1975 DAVID BALTIMORE, HOWARD M TEMIN and RENATO DULBECCO shared the Nobel Prize. Baltimore's research has contributed greatly to the understanding of the role of viruses in the development of cancer. They discovered the enzyme reverse transcriptase which can transcribe RNA into DNA without the involvement of DNA.

Dates in Infectious Diseases

1976   The first recorded case of Legionnaire's disease occurred in Philadelphia during an American Legion Conference. It is caused by a bacterium that was not identified until after the outbreak and is now known to be responsible for thousands of cases of pneumonia.

1976   The H2 blocker Tagamet (cimetidine) was introduced by the SmithKline Corporation. The treatment revolutionized peptic ulcer therapy.

1976   Ebola virus (named after the Ebola River in Zaire) emerged in Africa, in Sudan and Zaire. The first outbreak infected over 284 people, with a mortality rate of 53%. A second Ebola virus emerged from Yambuku, Zaire, Ebola-Zaire (EBOZ) later that year and had a mortality rate of 88%.

1976   MCNEILL'S *Plagues and Peoples* is published. He concluded that epidemics have profoundly shaped human culture and history.

1976   BARUCH BLUMBERG and D. CARLETON GAJDUSEK received the Nobel Prize for their discoveries concerning 'new mechanisms for the origin and dissemination of infectious diseases'. These mechanisms concern acute diseases where symptoms appear some time after the individual has been exposed to an infectious agent.

1976   Swine flu, initially isolated in New Jersey, led to a massive immunization program. However, contamination of vaccines produced Guillain-Barre syndrome in 100,000 people, killing 5%.

Dates in Infectious Diseases

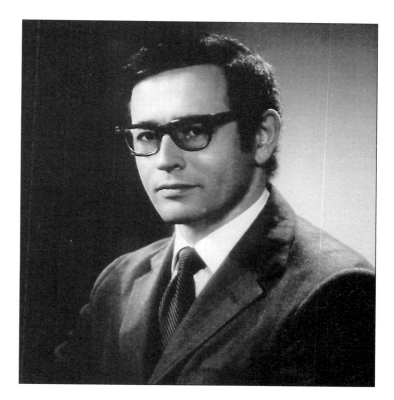

Gerald M. Edelman (b 1929)

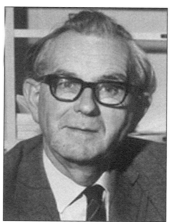

Rodney Robert Porter (1917–1985)

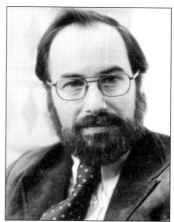

David Baltimore (b 1938)

Dates in Infectious Diseases

1977 — The parasite *Cryptosporidium* was linked to acute and chronic diarrhea parvum.

1977 — ROBERT AUSTRIAN completed development of a 14-valent pneumococcal vaccine.

1977 — CARL WOESE used RNA analysis to identify Archaea, a third form of life that is distinct from bacteria and eucarya.

1977 — *Influenza: The Last Great Plague*, was written by WILLIAM IAN BEADMORE BEVERIDGE, professor of anatomy and pathology at Cambridge University.

1977 — The last 'wild' case of smallpox was reported in Somalia. Two cases of laboratory infection were recorded in 1978. Smallpox is now considered eradicated. The total mortality attributed to smallpox in the twentieth century is 300–500 million.

1977 — JOSEPH McDADE and team isolated the bacterium that causes Legionnaires' disease. Further analysis revealed that the bacteria thrived in the cooling tower of the Bellevue-Stratford hotel. The first scientific account of the disease epidemic was given by DAVID WILLIAM FRASER, who named the bacterium *Legionella*.

1977 — WALTER GILBERT and FRED SANGER independently develop methods to determine DNA sequences.

1978 — Discovery of Hantaan virus, the cause of hemorrhagic fever with renal syndrome.

1978 — The United Nations adopted a resolution that set goals for eradicating infectious disease by the year 2000.

1978	Glaxo introduced the broad-spectrum injectable antibiotic Zinacef (cefuroxime).
1979	Identification of *Campylobacter* (now *Helicobacter*) *jejuni* as an enteric pathogen.
1980	On May 8, the World Health Assembly formally declared the world free of smallpox.
1980	Discovery of human T-lymphotropic virus 1 (HTLV-1), the cause of T-cell lymphoma–leukemia.
1980	Human interferon was produced in genetically engineered bacteria.
1981	Acquired Immune Deficiency Syndrome (AIDS) first gained recognition at the Center for Disease Control at Atlanta, Georgia. It is estimated that there are 34 million people living with HIV, 2.6 million deaths/year, and 5.6 million new infections/year.
1981	First vaccinations for hepatitis B.
1981	The anti-ulcer treatment Zantac (ranitidine) was launched by Glaxo and became the world's top-selling medicine by 1986. Augmentin (amoxicillin/clavulanate potassium) was launched by Beecham. The antiviral Zovirax (acyclovir) was launched by Wellcome for herpes infections.
1981	The bacteria which causes toxic shock syndrome was identified as a strain of *Staphylococcus aureus* by EDWARD KASS.

Dates in Infectious Diseases

1981 — Outbreak of Rickettsialpox in New York, caused by *Rickettsia akari*, transmitted among mice via mouse mites. Humans are incidental hosts.

1982 — Emergence of *Escherichia coli* O157:H7, the cause of hemorrhagic colitis and hemolytic uremic syndrome.

1982 — WILLY BURGDORFER of the National Institute of Allergies and Infectious Diseases isolated a previously unrecognized spirochete from the *Ixodes* tick, this was later named *Borrelia burgdorferi*.

1982 — JOHN VANE of the Wellcome Research Laboratories was awarded the Nobel Prize, with SUNE BERGSTRÖM and BENGT SAMUELSSON, 'for their discoveries concerning prostaglandins and related biologically active substances.'

1982 — Discovery of human T-lymphotropic virus ll (HTLV-ll), the cause of hairy cell leukemia.

1982 — STANLEY PRUSINER described prions.

1983 — The US mortality index attributable to infection was about 30 deaths per 100,000.

1983 — LUC MONTAIGNER and ROBERT GALLO announced the discovery of the human immunodeficiency virus (HIV) as the cause of AIDS. A test to detect the virus that causes AIDS was approved in the US.

1983 — Glaxo Inc launched the broad-spectrum injectable antibiotic Fortum (ceftazidime).

1983	*Helicobacter pylori* shown by BARRY MARSHALL of Australia to be the cause of peptic ulcers. This was the first infectious agent shown to cause a chronic disease that bears no features of an infectious disease.
1985	Tires imported into Texas from Asia carried larvae of the Asian tiger mosquito, a carrier of dengue fever and other tropical diseases. Within five years, Asian tiger mosquitoes were found in 17 States.
1985	The parasite *Enterocytozoon bieneusi* was found to cause persistent diarrhea.
1986	AZT (Zidovudine) was developed. The first antiviral agent to impact on HIV: 19 deaths in the placebo group and one death in the AZT group.
1986	KARY MULLIS established DNA polymerase chain reaction technology.
1986	Ehrlichiosis first described in the USA (although animal infections were described as early as 1935).
1986	*Cyclospora cayetanensis* was found to be a parasitic cause of persistent diarrhea.
1986	World scientists agree on a name for the AIDS virus: Human Immunodeficiency Virus, or HIV.
1987	The first fluoroquinolone was approved by the Food and Drug Administration in the USA. An intravenous formulation followed in 1991.
1987	The AIDS treatment Retrovir (zidovudine) was launched by Wellcome. Glaxo introduced the oral antibiotic Zinnat (cefuroxime axetil).

1988	Human herpes virus 6 (HHV-6) was identified. This causes roseola subitum.
1988	Hepatitis E, a type of foodborne hepatitis, was identified.
1988	An attempt to apply specific criteria and to define the illness 'myalgic encephalitis' (ME) was made by G.P. HOLMES and co-workers.
1988	SIR JAMES BLACK shared the Nobel Prize in medicine for his research into beta-blockers and the discovery of Tagamet. The co-recipients were GEORGE HITCHINS and GERTRUDE ELION of Wellcome, 'for their discoveries of important principles for drug treatment.'
1989	The cause of human ehrlichiosis, *Ehrlichia chafeensis*, was identified.
1989	SmithKline Beecham launched Energix-B hepatitis B vaccine (recombinant), a genetically engineered hepatitis B vaccine.
1989	Hepatitis C, a form of non-A, non-B hepatitis that causes liver infection, was identified.
1990	*Bartonella henselae* was identified as the cause of cat scratch disease, or bacillary angiomatosis.
1990	Rabies appeared in New York State raccoons. There were 2,746 animal rabies cases confirmed in the State in 1993. Between 1993 and 1995 human rabies deaths in the State were attributed to infection via bats. The World Health Organization 1992 figure for rabies deaths was 36,000 worldwide.

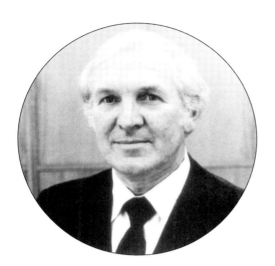

Sir James Black
(b 1924)

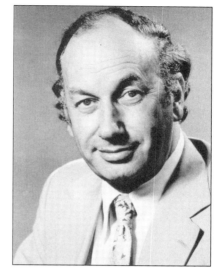

Sir John Robert Vane
(b 1927)

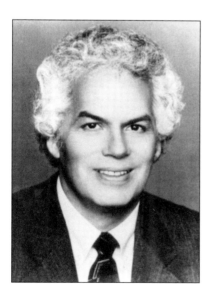

Stanley B. Prusiner
(b 1942)

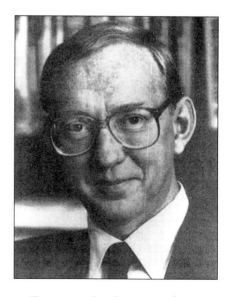

Bengt I. Samuelsson
(b 1934)

Dates in Infectious Diseases

1991   A major cholera outbreak occurred in Peru.

1991   Guanarito virus was shown to be the cause of Venezuelan hemorrhagic fever.

1991   MAGIC JOHNSON, the basketball star, announced that he was infected with HIV.

1991   The parasite, *Encephalitozoon hellem*, was associated with conjunctivitis and disseminated disease.

1991   A new species of *Babesia* was identified and found to be the cause of atypical babesiosis.

1992   DAVID GRAHAN show the effectiveness of antibiotic treatment on peptic ulcers. Thus finally confirming the involvement of *Helicobacter pylori*.

1992   A new strain of epidemic cholera, *Vibrio cholera* 0139, was identified.

1992   Mepron (atovaquone) for AIDS-related pneumonia was introduced by Wellcome in the US. SmithKline Beecham's Havrix hepatitis A vaccine, the world's first hepatitis A vaccine, was launched.

1992   *Tropheryma whippelii* was discovered and named as the cause of Whipple disease.

1993   Hantavirus outbreak in the Southwest USA. This was known as Si Nombre virus and causes adult respiratory distress syndrome. The disease is transmitted by exposure to rodent excrement and bites, and results in flu-like symptoms, severe respiratory problems, possible death. The virus is divided into two groups:

one found in Asia and Europe, the other in the United States.

1993 PAUL W. EWALD noted that pathogens either quickly evolve a counterdefense or become extinct. He suggested classifying phenomena associated with infection according to whether they benefit the host, the pathogen, both or neither.

1993 The World Health Organization declared tuberculosis to be a global emergency. Globally, one person is newly infected every second. Estimates put the expected death toll at around 35 million in the next 20 years.

1993 The parasite *Encephalitozoon cuniculi* was shown to be a cause of disseminated disease.

1994 A plague outbreak occurred in the summer in Surat, India following an earthquake in September 1993. There were 2500 cases reported and 855 deaths.

1994 The US mortality index attributable to infection rose to 60 deaths per 100,000. About half of these are attributable to AIDS, and the rest to respiratory disease, antibiotic resistance, and hospital-acquired infection.

1994 Sabia virus was shown to be the cause of Brazilian hemorrhagic fever.

1994 A National Institutes of Health Consensus Development Conference concluded that there is a strong association between *H. pylori* and ulcer disease, and recommended treatment with antibiotics.

Dates in Infectious Diseases

1994 — The Americas were declared polio-free. Polio-free zones also existed in Western Europe and in the Pacific basin, and by September 1995, 146 countries reported zero polio cases.

1995 — Neonatal tetanus deaths were 489,000, with 80% in only 12 countries.

1995 — Researchers from London and Glasgow provided evidence indicating that childhood diabetes is related to infection with Coxsackie B viruses. The researchers found the genetic material of Coxsackie viruses in blood samples from children at the onset of diabetes.

1995 — Hepatitis B vaccine now used in 28 countries as part of the routine immunization program.

1995 — Ebola virus outbreak in Africa. WHO reported that the Ebola virus appeared in Zaire in April. After two months, 93 infections and 86 deaths occurred. This 90% mortality rate is similar to an earlier Ebola outbreak in Zaire in 1976, where 290 died out of 318 people infected.

1995 — CRAIG VENTER, DAVID HAMILTON SMITH, CLAIRE FRASER and colleagues sequenced the complete genome of *H. influenzae*.

1995 — Valtrex (valaciclovir) was launched by Glaxo Wellcome as an anti-herpes successor to Zovirax (acyclovir).

1995 — About 33% of the world's population were estimated to be infected with tuberculosis: Britain 13% and the USA 7%. However, among the homeless in London, the rate was 25%, while among the homeless in San Francisco it was 30%.

1995	Human herpes virus 8 (HHV-8) was shown to be associated with Kaposi sarcoma in AIDS patients.
1996	PETER DOHERTY and ROLF ZINKERNAGEL received the Nobel Prize for their discoveries concerning how the immune system recognizes virus-infected cells. Their discovery has, in its turn, laid a foundation for understanding of general mechanisms used by the cellular immune system to recognize both foreign microorganisms and self molecules.
1996	The last two Americans to die of plague, both due to transmission by prairie dogs. Forty per cent of the US land area is infested by plague-infected animals, mostly prairie dogs.
1996	DAVID HAMILTON SMITH and PORTER W. ANDERSON were awarded the Albert Lasker Clinical Medical Research Award 'for visionary leadership in bringing the life-saving *Haemophilus influenzae* type b vaccine to a world market.'
1997	The avian flu H5N1 transferred to some Hong Kong citizens, a third of whom died. The Hong Kong health authorities destroyed 2 million chickens, and probably averted the possibility of worldwide spread of H5N1.
1997	Resurgence of diphtheria in Russia, where cases have increased from 2,000 in 1991 to 150,000–200,000 in 1997.
1997	An outbreak of hantavirus in Chile killed 25 people.
1997	A report describing a case of multiple antibiotic resistant bubonic plague was published. The causative agent, *Y. pestis*, acquired a resistance plasmid from an unknown source.

Dates in Infectious Diseases

1997 STANLEY PRUSINER, who first demonstrated that diseases such as bovine spongiform encephalopathy (BSE) and Creutzfeld–Jakob disease were caused by infectious proteins called prions, was awarded the Nobel Prize for Physiology or Medicine.

1998 ROBERT F. FURCHGOTT, LOUIS J. IGNARRO and FERID MURAD received the Nobel Prize for their discoveries concerning 'nitric oxide as a signaling molecule in the cardiovascular system.' NO produced in white blood cells is toxic to invading bacteria and parasites.

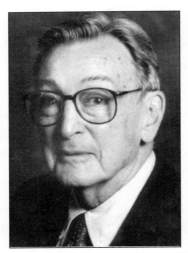

Robert F. Furchgott (b 1916)

1998 The worst outbreak of *E. coli* O157.H7 occurred in Wishaw, Scotland, with 500 cases and 20 deaths.

1998 SmithKline Beecham and the World Health Organization announced a collaboration to eliminate lymphatic filariasis (elephantiasis) by the year 2020.

1999 The malaria vaccine developed by ALTAF LAL of the Centers for Disease Control in Atlanta successfully passed its first tests.

Dates in Infectious Diseases

1999 The first drug against the killer bacterium, E.coli 0157 was developed in Canada. This has reduced hemolytic uremic syndrome which causes kidney damage.

1999 A new inhalational drug, Zanamivir, was approved to fight flu, blocking a viral enzyme called neuroaminidase, so preventing flu virus from escaping the cell.

1999 The first HIV vaccine trial in Africa began. This uses a weakened canarypox virus containing three HIV genes.

1999 JOSEF PENNINGER of the Ontario Cancer Institute showed that *Chlamydia* triggers an autoimmune disorder which can cause heart disease.

2000 The average life-span has lengthened to 77 years (74 years for males and 80 for females).

2000 In Malaysia, a new infectious entity, the Nipah virus, killed up to 100 people. The authorities destroyed a million livestock to help contain the outbreak.

2000 HARVEY ALTER and MICHAEL HOUGHTON were awarded the Lasker Prize for their work on hepatitis C and development of screening methods for transfusion-related hepatitis.

2000 New York was affected by bird- and mosquito-borne West Nile encephalitis, leading to widespread insecticide spraying. Mortality was only a few percent of those infected.